THE
COMPETITIVE
EDGE

THE
COMPETITIVE
EDGE

*The West Point Guide
for the Weekend Athlete*

by
Col. James L. Anderson
and
Martin Cohen

WILLIAM MORROW AND COMPANY, INC.
New York   1981

The views of the authors do not purport to reflect the positions of the Department of the Army or the Department of Defense.

Copyright © 1981 by Col. James L. Anderson and Martin Cohen

* * *

The illustrations on pages 187, 207, 226 and 228:
From Thompson, Clem W.: *Manual of Structural Kinesiology*, ed. 8, St. Louis, 1977, The C. V. Mosby Co.

The illustrations on pages 181, 182, 184, 185, 202 and 205:
Adapted from chart reproduced with permission of Cramer Products, Inc., P.O. Box 1001, Gardner, Kansas 66030.

The illustrations on pages 187 and 199:
Adapted from drawings reproduced with permission of Foot Control, Inc., P.O. Box 401690, Dallas, Texas 75240.

The illustrations on pages 201, 206 and 214:
Reprinted with permission from the book *The Doctor's Guide to Tennis Elbow* (etc.), by Leon Root, M.D. and Thomas Kiernan, copyright 1974. Published by David McKay Co., Inc.

Library of Congress Cataloging in Publication Data

Anderson, James Lee, 1933–
    The competitive edge.

    Includes index.
    1. Physical education and training. 2. Exercise.
3. Physical fitness. 4. Sports. I. Cohen, Martin
Aver, joint author. II. Title.
GV711.5.A52   613.7′1   80-23535
ISBN 0-688-00352-4

Printed in the United States of America

First Edition

1   2   3   4   5   6   7   8   9   10

BOOK DESIGN BY MICHAEL MAUCERI

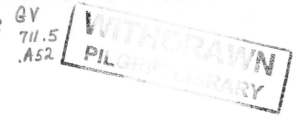
THIS BOOK IS DEDICATED TO

West Pointers who became great athletes, including:

the 2 James E. Sullivan Memorial Trophy Winners
the 3 Heisman Trophy Winners
the 98 who were members of U.S. Olympic teams
the 100's who were elected to All American teams
the 1000's of letter winners who went on to become great
weekend athletes

West Point athletes whose names are etched in history, including:

Douglas MacArthur	Creighton W. Abrams, Jr.
Dwight D. Eisenhower	James A. Van Fleet
Omar N. Bradley	Edward A. White
John J. Pershing	Joseph W. Stilwell
Lucius Clay	George S. Patton, Jr.

the great coaches who taught them, including

Earl "Red" Blaik	Herman J. Koehler
Vince Lombardi	Charles Daly
Bobby Knight	Biff Jones
Dr. Lloyd Appleton	Frank Diamond
Joseph W. Stilwell	Tom Jenkins
Morris Touchstone	Tom Cavanaugh
Joseph Palone	Garrison H. Davidson
Eric Tipton	

With special thanks to Lt. Col. Robert G. Tetu, Carol E. Tetu, Capt. F. L. Hagenbeck, and Judy A. Hagenbeck of West Point for demonstrating the exercises used in this book.

There's only one thing—
The joy of competition,
The joy in knowing you're ready
to go,
That you're the best person you
can possibly be at that moment . . .
                    —JOE PATERNO

        Pennsylvania State University
        Director of Athletics and
        Head Football Coach

Contents

The minute you sit back and don't want to compete whether it's in business, in medicine or in sports, on the golf course, on the tennis court, in swimming or whatever it may be—the minute you don't compete you start to sag, you get to be old, mediocrity sets in and you lose that zest for life.
—JOE PATERNO

Foreword

The Joys of Cooking, Sex, and Competition, An Unscientific Comparison

In the beginning it looked uncomplicated. We would write a hard-core text for the person who plays to win on the courts, the field and in the conference room. Tell this reader how to get a competitive edge and how to use it. And then a funny thing happened on the way to the publisher. Our basic premise was attacked on psychological and moral grounds.

It began with a phone call from the articles editor of a prestigious weekly magazine tendering an assignment. Subject: the psychological damage incurred by school children who participate in competitive sports. The idea had come out of the editor's personal experience. As a youngster she had been awkward and had found game participation embarrassing. Now her children, although doing well academically, were being "humiliated" in the school gym.

How did she know that her children were hurting?

"They lose a lot," she said. "That's bound to hurt a child."

How often did they lose?

"At least half of the time," she guessed.

Fifty percent isn't bad. In professional baseball, winning 50 to 60 percent is often good enough to win a pennant. Tennis pros win only 30 to 60 percent of their games. And Jack Nicklaus notes that in golf you need only a 20 percent win record to be among the best. In some competition the percentage is far lower. In the New York Marathon there were only two "winners" out of 12,000 participants.

19

The editor didn't think that adult statistics meant much to youngsters but there were several recent studies of children worth talking about. One was an examination of Little League teams in upstate New York to determine the effect of losing on children. The losing teams showed no depression, no psychological damage. In fact, the winning teams appeared to have a little anxiety which is not unusual because to the victors belongs the responsibility of defending honor and reputation.

Another study, out of Oklahoma, concluded that sports competition teaches youngsters to follow rules, hang in when losing, rebound from mistakes and work with others. However, none of these conclusions is in any sense remarkable. In the past several decades a great number of research projects have found athletic participation to be a great character builder although the kids themselves couldn't care less.

Of course, some youngsters have bad experiences in competition, but Dr. Charles Owens, a psychology professor at the University of Alabama, believes that the problem is more likely to originate with the parents or the coach. When his eight-year-old son announced his "formal retirement" from tennis, Dr. Owens studied the situation and discovered that it was his own fault, that he had put too much pressure on his son to win, and when he began to look around the ball parks he concluded that it was the "Little League Parent Syndrome" that was responsible for most of the emotional fallout among children.

The editor was politely attentive but it became clear that we had conflicting viewpoints. The conversation ended with our agreeing "to think about it," a courteous way of acknowledging two ships that were meant to pass in the night.

That was the season for consciousness raising, and so the editor's comments provoked a discussion the following weekend at West Point. In the end, we decided against defending athletic competition in the book, not out of arrogance but because the criticism appeared to be isolated. We were wrong. There were more brickbats on the way.

Within a week, a feminist friend published an essay in which she declared that athletic competition is "dehumanizing," and concluded that sports, especially football, are nothing more than a substitute for war or something that men do to pass the time while they are waiting for another war. That initiated a letter reminding the writer that athletic competition was originally formalized as a religious ceremony, a tribute to ancient deities. More recently, John Paul II has said that "sports competition is a commitment to seek the truest and most lasting victories—those of the spirit."

In fact, athletic competition was a major factor in the civilizing of man. The invention of the Olympics by the ancient Greeks was a cultural shock for other nations. The story is told of Xerxes, the Persian king, landing on Greek shores about 480 B.C. with an army of 20,000 men looking for a war. When he heard that the adult population was attending public games at Olympia, Xerxes sent a message pleading with the Greeks "to dispense with game playing and field an army."

Still, Xerxes was no more perplexed by athletic activity than contemporary critics. For example, a *New York Times* medical reporter, discussing how to avoid tennis elbow, writes about "tennis enthusiasts banging out their tensions on a small fuzzy ball" with the implications that the weekend athlete uses games to release hostility. And she misses the real danger—that using a bat, golf club, or racquet to discharge internal pressures may just as likely result in a stroke as a tennis elbow.

Perhaps the most devastating criticism was that of Tom Tutko, a psychologist and cofounder of the Institute of Athletic Motivation at San Jose State University, who describes athletes for the most part as being miserable and unhappy. Tutko notes that "most Americans truly believe that they're going to walk on water if they win. But winning is like drinking salt water. It's never satiable."

Tutko's description of the athlete is virtually identical with a psychiatric description of a "compulsive gambler" but the analogy doesn't work. The compulsive gambler lacks discipline, skills and training. Furthermore, the compulsive gambler expects to win something for nothing, in fact, for just being. On the other hand, the athlete knows he must pay the price.

In relating to criticism, you must always consider the source, and the next source was a surprise. We learned over the dinner table that one author's wife thought that most men play "like barbarians" —and she wasn't referring to professional football and hockey players but weekend players. The other wife then complained that she was treated as a barbarian by other girls because she was thought to be too aggressive in soccer games but had never had that problem when she played baseball or football with boys.

We went into conference again. We had been sensitized to the criticism, curious about the emotionalism and anger. Except for Tutko and Xerxes, most of the criticism came from women, who suffer from what sociologists call deprivation factors. One of the deprivation factors is that most women have been discouraged from getting into athletic competition. As a result, many don't know what they are talking about when they discuss sports.

We found support for this viewpoint in a statement from Penn State psychologist Dr. Dorothy Harris, who observes that all the traits that are "considered healthy psychological development in man (aggressiveness, independence, ambition, courage and competitiveness) are learned in the sports laboratory." She also used the words "deprivation factor" when talking about young girls who don't participate in sports. However, Dr. Harris notes that the enumerated traits are present in any athlete whether male or female.

Also, Stephen Rosenbloom, a psychiatrist and nationally ranked squash player, took issue with Tutko's conclusion that athletic competition is responsible for personality problems. Instead, Dr. Rosenbloom defines "the experience of competing and winning as a creative activity engaged in by a confident and complete self.'

Although athletic participation may not be a prerequisite for becoming President or a great scientist, the factor is usually there. George E. Vaillant, a psychiatrist at Harvard Medical School, found that participation in competition was a common trait in a study of 95 successful Harvard graduates, including captains of industry, scholars, cabinet members, physicians, and one U.S. President. Besides being high achievers, these men had happy homes and rich friendships. All of them were weekend athletes who played regularly with friends. Furthermore, Dr. Vaillant found that with maturity and success, these men became more active in competitive sports than they had been during their undergraduate years.

Such supporting studies and opinions of other professionals are relished when putting together an argument, but it doesn't mean much to the noncompetitor. None of these studies really answers the questions a woman put to her husband as they came off the courts after a session of mixed doubles.

The woman, obviously annoyed, asked, "Don, why do you have to hit the ball so hard?"

He didn't answer.

And then she buried him with a second question.

She asked, "What's so important about winning when you're playing with friends?"

You could tell from his eyes that he was already a thousand miles away, probably taking refuge in the thought that she would never understand. For her part, she will tell you that Don is one of the kindest men in the world until he gets into a game.

She says, "Give Don a racquet or any kind of stick and a ball and he turns into the Hulk."

Don is right. She doesn't understand. An emotional gulf exists between those who compete and those who don't, and it is often perplexing and disturbing. One weekend athlete, Bill Schutsky, a West Pointer, said that he found criticism of competition difficult to deal with.

He said, "Lots of people feel about competition as they do about religion, and if you hear negative talk at a party, if someone begins to bad-mouth sports competition, there's no sense in arguing about it. You just ignore it."

Schutsky was one of a number of weekend athletes interviewed, although the primary purpose was to learn their needs and problems in weekend competition. Most were men, but we also talked to over a dozen women, ranging in age from a 16-year-old who insisted that women could be both competitive and sexy to a middle-aged tennis player who remembered that as a teenager she wouldn't chance beating a date. And then there was Carol Tetu, who went more than thirty years believing that she was noncompetitive until her husband and sons talked her into running in a 10,000-meter road race.

She remembers, "I didn't think I had a competitive drive to win but after coming in second, I knew that I wanted to be first."

All of the adult interviewees held responsible positions and all had good educations—most had graduate degrees. They were chosen for selfish reasons because we wanted people who were intelligent*

---

* You don't have to be a genius to be a good athlete. On the other hand, being intelligent is no handicap. Intelligent people admire skills, learn them quickly, and can apply imagination to the job of winning.

and articulate. With only two exceptions, all described themselves as highly competitive. (Their spouses agreed and sometimes added "excessively competitive.") The two exceptions, both women, described themselves as "moderately competitive," whatever that may mean.

All insisted that sports was not the most important activity in their lives. Ahead of sports were family and work or academic pursuits. They talked about sports adding zest to their lives, but perhaps sports mean more. Most admitted that when injury or illness temporarily sidelined them, they became anxious about getting back. One began playing left-handed tennis while waiting for a broken right arm to heal. A topnotch athlete, the experience, nevertheless, reminded him to keep his eye on the ball.

Many of the interviewees were parents. Often they talked about the paradoxical situation of having one child who was very competitive in sports and another who was not. They all insisted that as parents they fully respected a youngster's preference for sedentary hobbies and interests.

The interviewers were never put on the defensive because they were competitive. Good journalism does not necessarily require giving people a hard time. When it came to subjective issues, they were merely encouraged to talk, and several interesting points were made.

The suggestion that the weekend athlete competes to discharge hostility was rejected. Without exception, all stated that they preferred to compete with people whom they liked and felt at ease with. These were friends, often very good friends, people whom they would not want to alienate.

When asked about sport celebrities they admired, most named athletes such as Chris Evert Lloyd because "she is ladylike" or Frank Gifford because he "behaves like a gentleman."

Most thought that the statement "winning is everything . . . or the only thing" was an unfair characterization of both weekend athletes and the national spirit.

And when we asked why they played with such intensity, they began to explain what it is that the noncompetitor doesn't understand.

All said that they prefer to play stronger and better opponents. Given a choice, they would choose to decrease their chance of winning by facing a more experienced and more successful opponent for several reasons:

—you can test your skills, endurance and nerves,
—you learn where you must improve your game,
—you are likely to learn something from your opponent's game,
—and, finally, to meet the greater challenge, you have to play at your very best. One said, "There's more satisfaction in losing a tough game than winning an easy game." It was this point that led to articulation of the subjective side of competition.

One weekender said, "When you are playing your best, drawing on all of your resources, you begin to feel a sense of exhilaration that is unique."

U.S. Senator Bill Bradley, former basketball star and Rhodes Scholar, in capsulizing his athletic career, said, "The real joy is playing."

In fact, the champagne and the trophy are anticlimactic. Eric Heiden said that he could do without the gold medals. And this is what the noncompetitor fails to understand—that even winning is anticlimactic.*

What counts is the act of competition, the striving to win, the testing of skills and nerve, endurance and spirit. And the greater the challenge, the tougher the match, the more exhilarating the contest. Sometimes it makes the question of winning purely academic, as Pete Rose noted in the 1975 World Series.

The sixth game of the Series was dramatic all the way as Boston and Cincinnati went past midnight into 12 innings. In the tenth inning Pete Rose, one of baseball's greatest competitors, came to the plate, turned to Sox catcher Carlton Fisk and said, "This has been such a great game that it doesn't matter who wins."

Although Cincinnati lost the game, it didn't change Pete's tune. Afterwards he was to say, "It has to be the greatest World Series game in history. I'm just glad to be able to say I was in it, and I'll be telling my son about it for a long time."

* Carol Tetu says that she can't understand why her husband and son make so much fuss about her trophies, and possibly there's an insight there. Trophies may mean more to friends, relatives and fans than to the actual winners—unless you are a professional negotiating a new contract.

His son would understand because the competitive experience isn't only for the pro or weekend athletes. Children feel it, too. In the community of Armonk, N.Y. where IBM has its headquarters, the parents run a soccer league for their children. On a Saturday before Thanksgiving, when the youngsters were playing for the league championship, the following conversation occurred between two eight-year-olds as they came off the field.

First boy, "You played a great game."

Second boy, "You did, too."

Hot, sticky, and exhausted, they paused for a moment to beam at each other, and then the conversation resumed.

First boy, "What was the score?"

Second boy, "I don't know."

Still grinning, they separated to find their respective coaches and learn who won.

To talk about the joy of competition is difficult for most Americans. We are a hardworking society that only in recent years has admitted to the joys of cooking, sex, and running. To suggest that sports competition also has a unique pleasure to offer other than building character or a healthy body may sound slightly blasphemous.

It's not likely that anyone will confuse the joys of cooking and sex, but the inexperienced may assume that the joys of running and competition are the same. Not so. Most of the weekend athletes that we talked to hate running and endure it only as a conditioning exercise. They find running so mechanical that they learn to use road time to think about their work. A self-described "intense competitor," Major George Cantlay, a West Point officer, believes that most so-called marathon runners are kidding themselves. In reality they don't have to beat anyone. He observes that in a marathon over 90% of the runners are socializing because only two or three runners have a chance of winning and everyone knows who they are. Also, some runners admit that running is a lonely experience, and others talk about having highs or a religious experience.

By contrast, most sports competition requires mental alertness, the development of agility and skills, and, more than anything else, constant reaction and readjustment to the opponent's game. Competition makes heavy demands on body, brain and spirit but is worth it.

Another West Point competitor, David "Pete" Gleichenhaus, as he turned 40, noted, "Some very special days when you're playing handball or tennis, and the competition is very tough, everything seems to go right. Your mind and body seem to be in perfect synchronization. And it feels so good that you think you'd like to do nothing else for the rest of your life."

We're not implying that athletic competition is all there is to life or that it should be the most important aspect of your life. And competition is not recommended as a substitute for the multiple joys of cooking, sex and running, but if you have tried these others, then perhaps you owe it to yourself to experience the exhilaration of sports competition. To experience this unique exhilaration, you've got to be a tough competitor, develop a competitive edge. And that's what the remainder of this book is all about.

The will to win has always been greatly overrated as a means of doing so. The will to prepare to win and the ability to prevent losing are of far greater importance.
—BOBBY KNIGHT
Indiana University
basketball coach

PART I

Sports Medicine: An Overview

What It Means to You

Chapter 1

What Sports Medicine Means to You, Including a 55-Second Quiz to Determine If You Want It

If you would rather win than lose, you should take advantage of the new sports technology.

Behind the men and women who set new athletic records is a team of professionals that includes orthopedic surgeons, biomechanists, exercise physiologists, psychologists, and athletic trainers. Behind this team is a field of research called sports medicine, which is giving us scientific information about the proper training, feeding, and use of the human body. The hard fact of the matter is that merely working at a sport, practicing and playing, doesn't fully prepare you to win.

We're discovering that world-class athletes who spend years preparing for an Olympic event may lose the gold not from a lack of effort, but from ignorance of the right kind of conditioning. For example, our Olympic basketball and volleyball players displayed excellent leg and aerobic strength, but upper-torso weakness blunted their ability to set up and spike the ball. Similarly our best swimmers, who are among the most conscientious athletes in the country, demonstrated upper-torso weakness, especially among the women, that limited their speed and endurance.

The professionals, whether their game is golf, tennis, basketball, football, baseball, or hockey, are beginning to realize that what separates them from the winner's trophy may be an imbalance of body composition, the lack of specific conditioning for a specific sport, or insufficient flexibility.

For world-class athletes, the scientific approach of sports medicine means new world records and the prestige of gold medals. For the pro, it's glory and a better contract. For the weekend athlete, who has limited time for conditioning, the new technology is a shortcut to getting a competitive edge.

Do You Need It? Do You Want It?
A 55-Second Quiz

Sports research begins with an analysis of what a sport demands of the body in movement, muscular strength and endurance, and cardiorespiratory efficiency and then prescribes a program to improve performance. That is what the book will do for you at the level of weekend competition.

Do you need it?

Originally we prepared a test of various muscle groups, but that didn't make sense if you happened to be looking this over in a bookstore or examining a friend's copy. Instead, we've prepared a quiz that you can take in the privacy of your head without moving a muscle or lifting your eyes from the page. Your answers should give you an idea of your fitness for recreational sports.

Q. After a weekend of your favorite sport do you dread the soreness that will follow you to work on Monday morning?

Q. When the outcome of a game is still doubtful and your opponent appears to be as strong as ever, do you find yourself losing your zest to win? Do you want to know why?

Q. World-class and professional athletes may spend a week or more preparing themselves mentally for a game. Would you like to know how to set yourself up in the 15 minutes it takes you to get from the office to the club?

Q. When you run for a ball or a bus, do you jiggle in the wrong places?

Q. Are you reluctant to play someone who is a better player? Do you know why you should overcome this attitude?

Q. Are you prone to suffer minor injuries? Achilles tendonitis? Low-back pain? Hamstring pulls? Other sprains and strains?

Q. Do you admire a tough competitor? Would you like to be a tough competitor?

Q. Would you like to know how correcting a problem as common and simple as pronation will improve performance and eliminate sore, tired feet?

Q. Would you like to know how to dominate a game? Or know what to do when you are being dominated?

Q. Would you like to know why body composition tells you

more about health and performance than body weight does?

Q. Do you know what to do when you find your concentration lagging?

Q. Our energy comes from three major sources: carbohydrates, fat, and protein. Would you like to know which fuel source is the most efficient? Which is the most digestible? Which is preferred by the brain and muscles?

Q. Would you like to know what and when to eat/drink before a game?

Q. Would you like to know when you should and shouldn't play hurt?

Q. Would you rather win than lose?

If you answer yes to the above questions, this book is guaranteed to become one of your most valued possessions. If you want to go a step farther, evaluate your flexibility, muscular strength, and endurance for a specific sport, we'll tell you how to go about that in the privacy of your home in the next chapter. First, we would like to call your attention to one of the most common errors in the thinking of people who play to win.

Winners Learn from Winners

Most weekend athletes believe that the secret of a great performance is technique, but no matter what the sport may be, technique is never a mystery. The correct grip, stance, swing, follow-through can be learned from the club pro, at a sport clinic, or from a syndicated feature in the newspaper. Jim Bouton, who won two World Series games with the help of a knuckle ball, confessed that he had learned the pitch from the back of a box of breakfast cereal.

Technique is rarely the secret of winning. Very simple reasoning proves this. Most of us compete at our own skill level, and therefore, we are evenly matched. When one competitor falls behind in a game, perhaps even comes apart, the problem 90 percent of the time is conditioning, the result of the winner's being in better condition. This is a fact. Accept it, just as you accept the knowledge that a 60-year-old athlete cannot compete on an equal level with a 24-year-old.

Champions know that they have worked hard to get where they are, but most know very little about the various factors that account for their attaining a competitive edge. From the time athletes enter scheduled competition, there is someone else thinking for them. For some, including gymnasts, tennis players, golfers, and swimmers, the guardianship may begin in preteen years, as young as age 6 or 7, and the practicing may be as much as eight hours a day.

The scheduled athlete has the help of a host of specialists or at least one person who represents a group of thinking aides who include coaches, trainers, consultants, physicians, and nutritionists. The guardian is thinking about the athlete's nutrition, wind, body composition, general and specific conditioning and may even be concerned about the quality of the star's mattress. Kenny Howard, assistant athletic director at Auburn University, told us that he observes football players when they are chatting in the department's lounge in order to identify those who don't know how to relax.

Who thinks for you?

Unless you're a head of state, no one thinks of the weekend athlete's fitness, and that's the gap this book fills. That is the book's reason for being: to guide and help you perform competitively at your chosen level of activity. Eventually you will have to take over, think for yourself, and adapt the information to your specific needs. And that's not a bad way to go.

Increasingly the intelligent person is learning that he or she alone is responsible for maintaining health and fitness. There is no doctor, no pill, no gimmick that can do a better job than the individual—when you have the proper information.

Today any athlete, weekend or pro, can develop a sound fitness program based on scientific research in nutrition, cardiorespiratory function, and exercise physiology.

Anything less is mindless.

Chapter 2

How to Use the Book

The weekend athlete doesn't require the same level of fitness as a pro or college athlete. In fact, the returns in conditioning are so small at the top level that it would be a waste of your time to work too hard. However, we're not suggesting that you won't have to put out.

University of Alabama Coach Bear Bryant has said, "Gimmicks are for losers. Work is for winners."

West Point's Red Blaik coined a sentence that has become a classic in sports literature: "You've got to pay the price."

These statements require no explanation for anyone who has succeeded in any human endeavor. Accomplishment requires effort. Conditioning is the same. Anyone who suggests otherwise is indulging in pure scam.

We have identified our readers as men and women who are competitors, who understand the joy of achievement. We also respect the fact that their main responsibility is to their profession. Therefore, the conditioning program has been designed to use your time at optimum efficiency. The program takes under thirty minutes a day and less than that once you get the hang of it. You have the option of expanding the program or eliminating it on days you are playing.

The program is based on functional conditioning, the actual use of the body rather than exercises that simply lead to a cosmetic effect. Cosmetic exercises, which are prevalent today, are considered a macabre joke among physiologists because they only prepare you to look good if you are in a coffin. Functional exercises, which take no more time, improve your coordination, poise, agility, power, endurance, and health. Of course, cosmetics are a bonus. Functional exercises get you looking good whether you are in a game or merely walking across a room.

35

When to Use the Book

The general conditioning, Part II, will maintain athletic tone year round between seasonal sports.

The conditioning for specific sports, Part IV, can be used to prepare and maintain conditioning for team and recreational games, for old favorites and new sports.

The book works equally well for singles, couples, and families no matter what their level of play. The novice prepares his muscles to learn and practice new skills, and the expert gains a competitive edge. The youngster improves his chances of making the school team, and the golden age golfer shaves strokes off his game. The specific conditioning may also be used to ensure the enjoyment of a vacation.

Just about the time winter resort ads remind you to make reservations, turn to "Skiing" (page 298) and "Ice Skating" (page 290) for preparatory conditioning and thereby prevent several days of muscular soreness while your body adapts to unexpected demands. When the snow begins to thaw, turn to "Golf" (page 278), "Tennis" (page 324) or whatever other warm-weather sport you fancy. If you are going underwater, turn to "Scuba Diving" (page 250). For climbing, look up "Climbing" (page 257). If you are getting back in the saddle for the first time in months, look under "Horseback Riding" (page 283).

It's that simple, that direct. Use the book as you choose—to play better, to feel and look better, or mainly to develop a winning edge.

The Book and Its Parts

The writers chose an ambitious goal—to produce the most comprehensive, valuable fitness book ever published for the general public. It can be used as a reference and as a manual. Still, the separate parts of the book are sharply defined.

GAF (General Athletic Fitness) is your power base, designed to keep you at a vigorous readiness level between seasonal sports and give you an edge in your professional, social, and sexual life. The conditioning is also carefully designed to protect you from the common strains and sprains that occur in most sports activities. We cannot emphasize strongly enough that GAF conditioning is the foundation for specific athletic conditioning.

The subtitle for GAF is "The Winner's Circuit" because it is adapted from the same circuit training used at West Point by cadets and faculty, men and women who range in age from late teens into the upper fifties.

SAF (Specific Athletic Fitness) is a small encyclopedia that identifies the specific muscle groups and cardiorespiratory level required in specific activities and the specific conditioning to have these factors. This is where you develop an additional edge, but again the section may be used as a practical tool to anticipate activities that you will get into during a vacation.

If you wish to evaluate your present fitness for a sport, the procedure is simple. Turn first to GAF, and determine at what level you can perform the conditioning exercises. You will quickly rate the state of your flexibility, muscular strength, muscular endurance, and cardiorespiratory efficiency. Follow the same procedure in SAF with the current sport you are playing.

The Psychological Edge. There is a totality of agreement in the sports world (and almost any other endeavor) that if you're not ready mentally, you're not going to win. Athletes are more frequently involved in win-lose situations than any other group, more aware of the importance of being mentally alert. When Arthur Ashe was a tennis instructor at West Point, he stressed the importance of concentration. He explained that when he appeared to be taking a nose dive during a match, winning the first set 6–2 and then losing the second 2–6, it was due to a loss of concentration. Fortunately it was usually a temporary lapse.

Sports competition may be the best school in the learning and practice of competitive psychology. This section includes practical advice for maintaining concentration, methods in preparing a game plan, avoiding pregame tension, playing under pressure, and other mind sets that concern the weekend athlete.

Body Parts—Their Care and Maintenance. We concluded that the thinking competitor would want to get under the skin and learn how muscles and bones work during sports activity, and so we discuss biomechanics in the context of steps that you can take to avoid strain and sprain, including the use of mechanical devices. However, accidents happen, and we know that competitors cannot abide being benched. They have an almost compulsive need to be active again. Therefore, we talk about first aid, when you shouldn't play hurt, and, most important, comeback conditioning.

West Point has led sports research in the prevention and treatment of injuries. A cadet's comeback conditioning begins as soon as the injury is diagnosed by a medical team. If the injury requires surgery, rehabilitation therapy usually begins before the cadet goes into the operating room.

Still, the question may arise: Why should West Point be your authority for fitness?

Chapter 3

Why West Point?

The public's perception of West Point's being a highly disciplined environment is correct. However, the Academy is not in the business of stifling either initiative or self-reliance. Just as cadets are individually responsible for meeting academic standards, each is responsible for maintaining physical standards. There is no first sergeant who orders cadets into the dawn's early light to engage in compulsory calisthenics.

The cadets have an advantage. Because West Point ranks as one of the world's best sports laboratories, cadets receive the most sophisticated conditioning information, which we will pass along to you. Each cadet must then act on this information just as you may choose to do.

You may further identify with cadets because they come to us with problems that are common to the general population. We get plebes who use their feet incorrectly when they walk and run, or have a deficiency in grip strength which is just as important in handling a rifle as a racquet or golf club. We even get former high school basketball and football stars who have surprisingly poor upper-torso strength. Also, we work with cadets who have never before held a racquet or golf club, and we know the problems of the novice.

West Point has more experience in the teaching and practice of recreational sports than does any other educational institution. West Point teaches lifetime sports to every student. The program is mandatory, scheduled like an academic subject, three to four times a week throughout the cadets' four years. Depending on their ability, cadets are required to compete at club, intramural, or collegiate levels. This gives West Point an exceptional overall experience in a range of sports activity that includes:

Aerobics	Mountaineering
Badminton	Orienteering
Baseball	Pistol
Basketball	Racquetball
Boat Racing	Rifle
Bowling	Rugby
Boxing	Sailing
Cross-Country	Scuba
Cycling	Skeet and Trap
Decathlon	Skiing
Fencing	Soccer
Flickerball	Softball
Football	Sport Parachute
Golf	Squash
Gymnastics	Strength Development
Handball	Swimming
Hockey	Tennis
Horseback Riding	Touch Football
Ice Skating	Track
Indoor Track	Triathlon
Judo	Unarmed Combat
Karate	Volleyball
Lacrosse	Water Polo
Marathon	Wrestling

Cadets are encouraged to develop lifetime sports for several reasons.

Sports and fitness should be inseparable because conditioning by itself becomes a bore. The joy of competition is the payoff for conditioning. In our childhood we depend wholly on games to develop fitness and health. When parents tell children to go out and play, they are not thinking of checkers. Parents are correct in expecting children to benefit from games. However, as we get into the sedentary adult world, we learn that we must get fit in order to participate in sports. By encouraging cadets to develop lifetime sports, we are supporting a lifetime fitness program. One feeds the other.

Another reason behind the Academy's sports activity is solely concerned with the competitive spirit. During World War I Gen. Douglas MacArthur concluded that sports competition in itself develops such qualities as courage, leadership, and initiative, the same conclusion that psychologists have made since. When Mac-Arthur took over the post of superintendent at the Academy in 1919, he initiated a sports program as a major part of the curriculum.

At the Academy today there are four categories of education: academic, physical, moral/ethical, and military. Cadets must maintain high standards in all four. Obviously it would be intolerable if a large part of the cadet population suffered injury or undue fatigue in the physical activity required by military training and sports. As a matter of necessity, if for no other reason, West Point has emerged as an uniquely experienced practitioner of the science of developing endurance and strength and preventing athletic casualties.

Maintaining cadet fitness is the responsibility of the Physical Education Department, which is made up of fifty-two men and women, all of them specialists with graduate degrees engaged in sports research and education. In addition, the department includes visiting professors from other institutions and other recognized authorities who are consultants. As a result, West Point is frequently the site of Olympic training and meetings of various high-level committees on fitness, including the President's Council on Physical Fitness and Sports.

West Point's fitness experience with men goes back over 150 years. Depth research of American women's fitness began four years prior to their admission to the Academy and has included the study and testing of several thousand women. In the beginning of this research we were attacked by two different camps: the Neanderthals, who thought women should literally stick to their knitting, and the active feminists, who insisted that women can do anything that men can do and still have babies.

We have tended to side with the feminists, although we exclude West Point women from participation in football, wrestling, and lacrosse because of their obvious physical disadvantage in weight and muscular development. Some feminists disagree with these exceptions, but the vision of a 230-pound male crashing into a female quarterback or slamming a woman wrestler to the mat makes us shudder. The injuries would be appalling.

Still, we should note that for the past seven years women's fitness and conditioning have been among our major concerns. American women generally have been more feminine than feminist in their attitude toward sports activity, and this has resulted in their fitness's being neglected. These deficiencies show up when women apply for admission. To overcome these problems, West Point, in consultation with the nation's outstanding authorities on women's physiology, has developed the best women's fitness program in the world.

The above information is not hype. To the contrary, for the authors have become a little too sensitized by the extravagant claims made in many fitness books. Still, it is an overt effort to assure you that West Point is sophisticated in the whole spectrum of fitness—from preventive to comeback conditioning for general and specific conditioning, from the novice to the expert, and for men and women. The information in this book applies equally to both sexes with an occasional footnote that may be helpful to those who are entering the sports arena for the first time.

Be further assured that the conditioning programs in this book have been carefully designed to bring you along gradually, to improve your performance and endurance progressively without discomfort, injury, and undue fatigue.

What follows is an overview of sports medicine today. However, it's something more than a review of achievements. We believe it will give you a substantial perspective on fitness as it relates to your own needs.

Chapter 4

The Mystery of the Disappearing Muscles

Maj. Denny Leach, in his mid-thirties, has always kept himself fit. He is five eleven and trim with good shoulders and muscular body. He looks like a good weekend athlete, which he is. When Leach came up to West Point for a three-year tour, he was encouraged to run because of his family's history of cardiovascular disease.

Always a competitor, Leach began to race and worked himself up to qualify for the Boston Marathon. He completed the 26 miles plus in under three hours, felt good about it, and also felt particularly strong and fit. And so the following week he decided to get around to beating "the old man," Jim Anderson, who plays a boss game of racquetball.

Leach, a genial kind of guy, approached Anderson and said amiably, "Colonel, I was hoping that if you have the time to play some racquetball with me, I'd get an idea of how well I'm coming along," which translates into: "Sir, I'm going to whip your tail."

Anderson, who translates quickly and is Leach's senior by ten years, stretched his old bones and graciously noted that he could use a workout, which translates into: "Major, I'm going to chew you into little pieces."

Being highly competitive is a way of life for most West Pointers for several reasons. First, like other colleges with high admission standards, West Point begins with a student body of high achievers. Then it is the policy at West Point to sharpen the competitive edge with compulsory year-round participation in sports. General MacArthur initiated the program with the policy "Every cadet an athlete." Colonel Anderson extended the policy statement to: "Every cadet an athlete, every cadet challenged," which means all cadets play at their highest level (club, intramural, varsity, world-class—depending on their abilities). And then, you see, Leach worked on Anderson's staff, and when Anderson screens personnel for the Academy's Physical Education Department, he selects assistants for their "lean and hungry look."

Leach met Anderson on one of the racquetball courts during lunch hour the next day. Anderson barely dredged out a win in the first game. In the second, Leach began to slow down, and Anderson won by a two-to-one margin. In the last game Leach was sluggish and lost badly.

Leach was let-down. Baffled was more like it. Why had he lost? He had proved his strength and endurance in the strenuous run at Boston, but back in the gymnasium he had nearly collapsed in less than an hour on the court. One onlooker guessed that Leach was having a "relapse" from all that conditioning for the marathon. He had "gone weak." That's impossible. Conditioning cannot be lost in a few days. Strength and endurance don't suddenly disappear.

Leach's experience is far from being unique. Similar experiences strike professional athletes who occasionally decide to take a wing at a recreational game. For example, a professional football star who loved high school basketball goes down to the neighborhood court to play pickup with friends. In twenty minutes he's dragging. He's dumbfounded by the unexpected fatigue. The pro will then argue that you can't be good at more than one sport at a time. That's a myth, too.

What happened to these two men?

Leach's cardiorespiratory conditioning was excellent, far more than he would need in an hour of racquetball. His problem was muscle fatigue, although it wouldn't make sense if you looked at Leach because his body shows muscle definition. However, in the fine tuning for the Boston Marathon he had stopped using the muscles in his upper torso and had overspecialized the conditioning in his legs.

In a 26-mile run, energy must be used most efficiently, conserved for the legs while the upper torso draws a bare minimum of oxygen and other nutrients from the blood. In effect, Leach had put his upper torso at rest for about three months while he was preparing for the marathon.

Furthermore, Leach's muscles were so painful after an hour of racquetball that he had trouble sleeping for two nights. Surprisingly the soreness extended down through the lower torso and into his legs. Why should this happen when his legs had worked so hard for several months?

Again, the efficiency of the long-distance runner depends on putting one foot down after another in a straight line. The handball court requires agility and many different combinations of leg and torso muscles.

The football player also had sore muscles because his line position doesn't require anywhere near the agility used in basketball, but what the lineman found a little scary was his getting winded so quickly in a few minutes of basketball. Well, that's another difference between football and basketball. About two-thirds of the time on a football field are spent in rest. This does not build up cardiorespiratory endurance.

There are several things wrong with the thinking of some athletes. As kids they played at a variety of sports with no problems, so they begin to think that if you're strong, you can play anything. When they begin to specialize in college or as pros, they find that if they play at another game, they hurt. They reason that it's impossible for them as specialists to handle another sport mentally or physically. They are totally wrong. Their reasoning is unscientific.

What we have learned from sports technology is that there's specific conditioning for every sport, and with specific conditioning you can go from one sport to another simultaneously or seasonally with success and pleasure. Or you can do it the hard way.

A woman runner finished her first competitive season by accepting an invitation from her husband to play some racquetball, a game that she really enjoyed. She looked forward to it as a change of pace. She had the same experience as Leach, including lots of pain for a couple of weeks. Her response was that she would rather go through the pain barrier than put up with conditioning. That's a choice, but then you end up with only minimal preparation— too little to gain a competitive edge and play a winning game.

If you'd like a moment to mourn the passing of the natural athlete, if you think that the natural athlete is another victim of modern technology, forget it. The natural athlete has been an anachronism for more than 2,000 years.

Sports Medicine—The Greeks Had the First Word, "Bull"

A number of stories are told about Milo of Crotona, a Greek athlete who was thought to be the strongest man in the world in the sixth century B.C. Milo was victor six times at the Pythian Games and six times at the Olympic Games.

According to one legend, Milo began to develop his strength as a youngster by carrying a newborn calf on his shoulders every day. After four years he carried the animal into the arena. Fully grown, it should have weighed a ton or more. That's a lot of bull, especially for a youngster to tote on his back, but it was to mark the end of barnyard conditioning. Milo was among the last of the world's self-made sport heroes.

By the fifth century B.C. athletes who hoped to compete in the Olympics were required to train for periods of up to ten months, observe strict diets, carry out specific exercises, and take an oath that they would obey the gymnasts, as trainers and coaches were called. Competitors were told, "If by your work you have been rendered worthy to go to Olympia, if you have not been idle or ignoble, then go with a good heart. But let those who have not trained in this fashion go where you will." Simply, shape up or ship out.

In ancient Greece athletic fitness was part of the concept of the whole man. A youngster's day was divided into three parts—academics, physical fitness, and rest. The concept of the whole person produced some of history's great philosophers, artists, poets, scientists, and political theorists.

The Greek concern with athletic fitness was partly based on the understanding that physical conditioning was not only good preventive medicine but also basic to a high degree of performance in all activities. So concurrently there was the birth of modern medicine and sports medicine.

About 400 B.C. Herodicus was the first to be concerned with diet and therapeutic exercise for both athletes and sick patients. His student Hippocrates recommended exercise for physical well-being and for mental disorders, just as some "running psychologists and psychiatrists" do today. Still, if Hippocrates is celebrated as the father of modern medicine, Herodicus deserves to be called the father of sports medicine because he was the first to recognize that athletic conditioning depends on the science of medicine.

Contributions of the ancient Greeks include:
- —The invention of protective devices such as ear guards and knuckle wrappings for boxers.
- —The use of hydrotherapy, weights, and pulleys in medical rehabilitation.
- —The advocacy of exercise therapy for heart disease accompanied by heart failure.
- —The introduction of medical massage before and after training by Iccus, also a winner of the pentathlon.
- —The recommendation of exercise during convalescence.
- —The description by Philostratus of body builds necessary for specific activities.
- —The advent of the "first team physician," Galen in the second century A.D.

Galen, one of the most brilliant men in medicine, was probably the first true exercise physiologist. He recognized that muscles have only one action—contraction—and wrote about the antagonistic action of different muscle groups. He introduced comprehensive physical examinations and the taking of medical histories. For about six years he was surgeon to the gladiators at Pergamum, where he predictably increased his knowledge of anatomy. As a result of this experience, he was publicly to condemn gladiating as a sport.

The ancient experts were often in conflict over training methods. Plato thought Herodicus was too zealous in prescribing exercise, and Hippocrates took issue with some aspects of specialization. Physicians prescribed diets to increase strength and sexual potency, but other physicians charged them with quackery. Public controversy was common, but then we must remember that ancient Greece was also the cradle of democracy.

The Greeks were brilliant but limited. If Milo, the greatest athlete of ancient Greece, had played an hour game of handball, he would have ended up with more pain than Major Leach, and what's more, he'd probably have fallen over himself and cracked a bone. Milo was muscle-bound, and being muscle-bound is no myth.

Chapter 5

Have Twitch, Will Travel—Analyzing Skills

The Greek concept of medical fitness was to rule for 1,000 years, until the Renaissance and the advent of chemotherapy with its medicine cabinet loaded with pills and drugs as if man had returned to magic potions and alchemy.

Although pill dependency is still a problem for many, early in the nineteenth century a Swedish poet, Pehr Henrik Ling, founded a gymnastic movement that swept through Europe and into America. Fitness was further promoted during the Napoleonic Wars by political leaders who recognized that national survival depended on good health.

What we now call sports medicine got its impetus in 1910 with a two-volume work, *Hygiène des Sports*, by a Berliner, Dr. Siegfried Weissbein. In 1913 the First International Congress on Sports Therapy and the Physiology of Exercise was held in Paris, and this marked the birth of modern sports medicine. Today, in Western Europe, students graduate from medical schools with degrees in sports medicine. In communist nations, sports medicine has been institutionalized in the hope that sports supremacy will be interpreted as political supremacy.

In the United States we have the President's Council on Physical Fitness and Sports and the American College of Sports Medicine, founded in 1954, with more than 5,000 members, including cardiologists, orthopedists, exercise physiologists, psychologists, psychiatrists, surgeons, coaches, podiatrists, nutritionists, and biomechanists. Within the nation an increasing number of medical schools and physical education departments, including West Point's, are involved in sports research.

Sports medicine is not limited to what's best for the Olympic athlete. The American concept includes study of exercise and recreational sports for the healthy and for those who are not, for those who are mentally or physically disadvantaged, and the programming of exercise programs and the prescription of nutrition to maintain basic physical fitness.

Sports medicine is the fastest growing specialty in the medical world and has already made a major contribution to the health of the general population. Still, it should be noted that sports medicine, like any other science, is corruptible. West German scientists report that Russians and East Germans are continuing to experiment with doping to improve competitive performance. For example, the Russians and East Germans not only continue to force large doses of anabolic steroids on their athletes but have also developed methods to prevent detection by normal testing standards.

Also, in Russia and East Germany, young children, some no more than 5 or 6 years of age, are "conscripted" into sport institutions to be trained and conditioned for future Olympic competition.* The next step, logical from a totalitarian viewpoint, is the breeding of athletes. None of this comes as a surprise during this century, when nations have used the Olympics to project an image of racial or political supremacy. It is simply explained by scholar J. M. Fulbright as "the totalitarian concept that the end justifies the means."

Conversely, responsible advocates of sports medicine in Western nations denounce doping of athletes as being morally wrong (cheating) and further note that such drug use is injurious to the athlete. The conscription of children is totally inimical to both democratic ideals and the concept of the whole man. Of course, there are athletes in Western nations who use drugs and cheat in other ways, as there are parents and guardians who push children into specialization, but these are instances of individual choice and individual corruption, not national policy.

Writing about corruption may be a digression, but we have tried to keep it short, and it's not a bad transition. It tells us that in world-class competition, where most of the research goes on, the gold medals will be won by those who are best able to take ad-

* Renate Vogel, a world champion swimmer before she defected to West Germany, has said that her doping (steroids and cortisone) to build muscle tissue began at the age of 9.

vantage of technological advances and genetic analysis. Although it's a whole new ball game, ironically we continue to deal with the same basic questions.

Are Winners Born? Made? Reborn?

Coaches have always looked for physical types. In selecting wrestlers, the ancient Greeks believed that bigger was stronger. Today basketball coaches look for tall men, and football coaches look for ancient Greek wrestlers. However, eye judgment is crude and primitive.

If you were checking inherited characteristics today, you would test a person for maximum oxygen intake, pulmonary ventilation, vital capacity, forced expiratory volume, and residual volume. And then "Doc" Counsilman, Indiana University's famous exercise physiologist and swimming coach, sorts out athletic talent with a simple test * for fast twitch muscle fiber.

Fast-twitch fibers are high in gylcolytic activity or anaerobic activity. Those who jump highest have the highest ratio of fast-twitch fiber and become the sprinters and short-distance swimmers.†
The slow-twitch fibers are better able to oxidate energy, and their possessors thereby become prime performers in long-distance and endurance events. Those athletes who have difficulty jumping over an egg without breaking it become candidates for the long-distance events. The mid-range jumpers are middle-distance runners and swimmers.

Each of us has a unique mixture of slow-twitch and fast-twitch muscle fiber, and it is genetic. Many sports scientists believe that black athletes dominate games that require speed because they are genetically endowed with more fast-twitch muscle fiber. And whites dominate long-distance events because they have a higher ratio of slow-twitch muscle fiber.

* Doc Counsilman uses the simple Sergeant's Jump, a jump-and-reach test. The person stands sideways with shoulder against the wall, feet flat and one arm stretched as high as possible, and the reach is marked. Next, and with only one try, he jumps as high as possible and is marked. The athlete with the most fast-twitch muscle fiber should jump the highest. *Note*: Use chalk dust or wet the fingertips to leave a mark on the wall at highest point of the jump.

† Also, the best receivers in football. They leap like birds and run like rabbits.

Still, the competitive edge doesn't necessarily go to the man with a genetic advantage. There are still the matters of motivation and conditioning. Reports from East Germany tell us that some youngsters chosen for their genetic superiority resist conditioning, and rather slyly. They hold back achieving conditioning goals because that means they will then have more advanced goals. Advanced goals require more work and also open the possibility of failure, and with failure they are no longer genetic elitists.

When you get to the bottom line of sports medicine, the magic words are "biomechanical efficiency." At the Munich Olympics, Russian sprinter Valery Borzov, winner of two gold medals, was offered as an example of an athlete who had been made biomechanically efficient.

Genetically Borzov was known to have good strength and speed, but certainly not the great speed of the American sprinters. However, he was trained to make every movement as mechanically efficient as possible. This included stride length, foot placement, body posture, and arm swing. Even his start was studied and improved. In short, the Russians took a good sprinter and made him into a great sprinter.

Although the American sprinters had the potential for great speed, they were thought of as born sprinters. They were not using their superior, natural talents as efficiently as Borzov was taught to use his. Why? Because at that time our coaches believed that the fastest sprinters were born, not made. Now that our coaches are spending more time correcting mechanical deficiencies, new sprinting records are assured.

Biomechanics is not a matter of tinkering with your body as if it were a piece of machinery, but a clinical study to learn where you have gone wrong and picked up some inefficient body movements, incorrect foot or arm placement, and stressful posture. And with biomechanical efficiency you get some aesthetics in almost any activity. You can enjoy the incredible grace and coordination of baseball player Graig Nettles fielding a ball and the biomechanical efficiency of a striptease dancer who knows exactly where to place her anatomy at any given moment.

For the weekend athlete, biomechanical efficiency is a Christmas gift from sports medicine. It is the key not only to better performance but also to the elimination of much strain and injury.

For example, if you apply mechanical analysis to the simple art of walking and running, you learn that proper foot placement is not this:

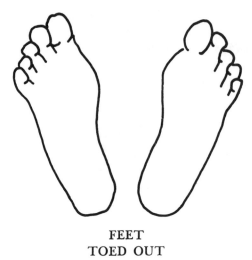

**FEET
TOED OUT**

and not this:

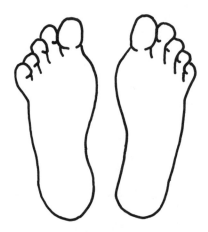

**INSIDES OF
FEET
PARALLEL**

but this:

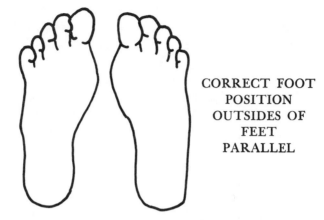

CORRECT FOOT
POSITION
OUTSIDES OF
FEET
PARALLEL

As the sketch illustrates, it is the *outside* of each foot that should fall on two parallel lines with a slight pigeon-toed look. Incorrect placement, with the toes pointed out or the insides of the feet parallel, not only wastes energy but risks injury to the feet and knee joints.

Biomechanics is the study of the biological activity, especially muscular, of the body in performance. To analyze the forces that act on the body and the effects that the forces produce, biomechanical techniques include the application of the laws of physics associated with projectile motion, elastic impact, Newton's laws of motion and their angular analogues, mechanical energy, center of gravity, buoyancy, and flotation and fluid resistance.

And that's also how we learn that running downhill exerts four times the body weight on feet, explaining why "the bones," if not the lungs, feel better running uphill.

West Point has been at the forefront in the study of biomechanics because the cadets may be the most physically active college student body in the world. On an average day a cadet puts as much as six strenuous hours into sports and military training. And like the weekend athlete, he works and plays in a highly competitive environment. And so back to the question: Is a winner born or made?

The answer has to be "made."

Although the cadets are a select group of high achievers academically and athletically, aggressive and competitive, they have a lot to learn about general fitness and athletic fitness. Besides military posture, they learn athletic posture—how to place their feet, move their torsos, and use their arms—and that's biomechanics. Without this expertise, even a genetically superior athlete may be a loser.

And are athletes reborn?

Yes. Rehabilitation of the injured athlete is another area in which West Point has pioneered, and here, too, is invaluable information for the weekender who has been either hurt or leading a sedentary life.

Perhaps none of these answers was unexpected, but here is a question that gets a lot of discussion in the locker room and the lab: What is more important to winning, psychological or physiological conditioning?

Two Major Factors Compared

In any year of sports there will be a number of upsets with the underdog defeating the odds-on favorite. This is illogical, much like a balloon defying gravity. We try to explain this away by observing that the losing team was overtrained or overconfident and that the underdog was hungry or tried harder. Was it the psychological or physiological factor that made the difference?

Some colleagues insist that the ultimate limit of performance is bound by emotional involvement. They talk about the "will to win" being the key to victory, but that appears to depend more on the level of competition. Although there's no scientific proof, and probably never will be, the psychological factor appears to be decisive at the highest level of competition—the Olympic level, in which the athlete reaches the highest level of conditioning. Perhaps this is best exemplified by the Roger Bannister story.

Until 1954 running the mile in under four minutes was considered a nearly impossible feat for a human. Some observers warned that a man's heart might burst in the attempt. In a century of recorded time the world's best runners hovered just above four minutes. And then an Oxford medical student, Roger Bannister, came along in May 1954 and broke the four-minute barrier. A month later John Landy, an Australian, broke Bannister's record. In August 1954 Bannister ran again and beat both his own record and Landy's. Now, in the 1980's, at any one time there are more than a dozen runners who can run the mile in under four minutes. What Bannister truly overcame was the psychological barrier.

Although the psychological factor is as important as the physiological for the finely tuned competitor, this is not true of most other athletes. The public usually overrates the conditioning of the professional and other scheduled athletes. At these levels of competition, being up for a game means being up physically as much as psychologically.

These are judgments that you are free to dispute of the mix at several levels:

> World-class level: 50% physiological,
> 50% psychological.
> Professional level: 60% physiological,
> 40% psychological.
> College level: 70% physiological,
> 30% psychological.
> Weekend level: 80% physiological,
> 20% psychological.

Despite the ratio in favor of fitness, we don't intend to de-emphasize the psychological edge. One big weakness in the weekend athlete's profile is not knowing how to set himself up mentally before a game. Other big problems include coping with too much pressure and too little concentration. Nonetheless, winning is obviously dependent on both major factors. In the final analysis, the most important aspect of confidence derives from being physically ready. Now exactly what is physical fitness?

Chapter 6

The Fitness Profile: Fit for What?

Lecturing around the country, one basic question comes up frequently with slight variations:

"Am I physically fit if I play tennis three times a week?"

". . . play golf every time I get a chance?"

". . . run three mornings a week?"

". . . play handball twice a week?"

The question is intelligent, an advance in the understanding of fitness. In the past most people concluded that anyone who picked up a racquet or golf club, wore sneakers or a running suit was physically fit. That's wrong. An avid golfer is likely to score low in cardiorespiratory fitness, and a person who plays only tennis isn't all that much better off. On the other hand, a person who regularly runs a half hour with poor posture is just a short time away from pain and an orthopedist. Similarly, a Hollywood star who does fifty push-ups and fifty sit-ups a day is getting cosmetic results. The sit-ups keep his stomach flat, and the push-ups condition his machismo.

At the core of this misunderstanding is the belief that physical fitness is a dichotomy, that you're either fit or not fit. And that's wrong. You cannot dichotomize fitness into contradictory parts as you do good or evil, dryness or wetness. In reality, physical health ranges from those in very poor health, unable to work or move about, to those in excellent health, who function freely with an absence of disease or symptoms. Fitness for physical activity ranges from the ability merely to flick an eyelid to the optimum level of a superior world-class athlete. To understand fitness, never think dichotomy because fitness is a continuum.

Life Is a Bowl of Continua

Most of life's activities, mental or physical, are continua. We know that we can improve our work performance, knowledge, physical and social skills. We learn that improvement itself is a continuum, a gradual development. No one goes from novice to expert overnight. Therefore, we must make decisions about the level of performance we wish to reach and maintain.

What this comes down to is individual choice and evaluation of our needs and desires—what we want for ourselves in terms of career, advanced educational, social, sexual, and athletic activity. "How much fitness?" then becomes a very personal question.

Fit enough to get through a day at work?

Fit enough after a day's work to go on to evening classes—or a concert, dance, party?

Fit enough to get up the morning after and put in a good day's work?

Fit enough to play a vigorous game at the end of the day?

Fit enough to be a tough competitor in that game?

The range of choice in fitness is further illustrated in the continuum triangle.

The diagram indicates the relative amount of work necessary to reach different levels of fitness, but important to remember is that with a rise in fitness you also have a rise in stamina, strength, and other components that improve performance and health. Fitness produces strength/performance, which in turn increases fitness and so on in an upward spiral. It is a beautiful option of nature, there for the individual's taking and use.

There's a direct correlation between the level of fitness and conditioning as long as the program is soundly conceived. On the other hand, if you follow such popularized recommendations as wiggling your toes when watching television or standing every time the phone rings, you won't do much for your cardio-respiratory or your skeletal muscles. You will only learn to rise at the ring of the bell instead of salivating like Pavlov's dog.

As noted above, the level of fitness is directly correlated with

PHYSICAL FITNESS CONTINUUM TRIANGLE

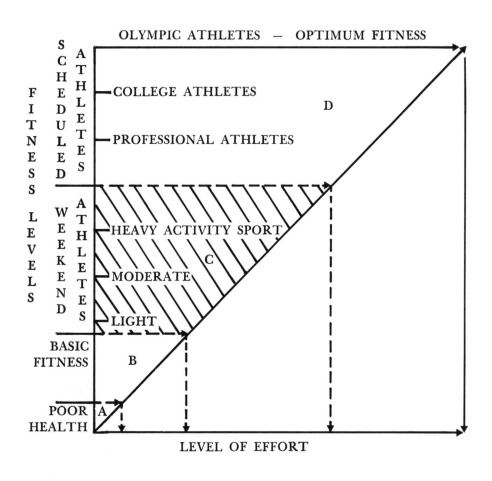

EFFORT INCLUDES:

— TIME
— INTENSITY
— COACHING
— (SKILL)

the level of effort that the person expends. The level of effort is defined by three components:

1. The amount of time that you can devote to your workout.

2. The intensity of your workout, or how hard you work during the conditioning.

3. The quality of the advice that is available to you. This would depend on the qualifications or the expertise of the trainer/coach or the book.

At the top of the continuum triangle, optimum fitness is represented by a broken line because there is no recognized limitation on conditioning or attainment. The human being continues to dazzle us with new levels of achievement in the sciences, philosophy, technology, sports, and other areas of challenge. Perhaps, like the universe itself, man's destiny is infinite. However, the base of the triangle is another story and a grim one. Below the base line is the absence of life, activity, and fitness.

Poor Health, Area A. Most of the people who fall into Area A are basically "breathers." They get out of bed to attend to a job. A bus, train, or car carries them to their work chair. They get up to have lunch, go home, and then walk from the dining table to the chair in front of TV and get up once more to go to bed. They are involved in the least possible amount of physical activity.

At the A level of fitness, a person is borderline, not really sick and not really well. He usually has chronic complaints about tension, headaches, insomnia, or body pains. Although the person functions on the job or in the home, this can be tipped downward easily with a slight infection. With illness, the breather goes to a doctor for a cure, takes medication, and eventually returns to the same substandard state of health.

Most of these people have been functioning at a substandard level of health for so long that they accept their condition as a natural state of health. Physicians seldom explain otherwise. Most doctors are fully occupied practicing curative medicine. The odds are against physicians' recommending health raising through a fitness program. The reason—doctors have become frustrated asking patients to stop smoking, overeating, overdrinking, etc.

When a person is run-down, a physician may recommend a

vacation, a rest, or a visit to a health spa, but this brings only temporary relief, a period of convalescence with little or no physical activity. This reinforces the idea that doing little or nothing is good for you when the individual should be treated like an injured athlete who is immediately drawn into a program of comeback conditioning. Instead, after a vacation the breather reverts to the same low level of physical activity. The breather's philosophy is simple: If you're sick, see a doctor; if you aren't sick, take aspirin, sleep pills, tranquilizers, anything that will help you get through the day, but do nothing that requires physical exertion.

At the top level of Area A you may have a person who is becoming aware that good health is an individual choice. The individual may be cutting down on smoking and drinking and be moving from diet fads to fitness gimmicks. Here the problem is ignorance: the man who walks a couple of miles to work and back but is grossly overweight; the woman who takes up a fashionable diet and finds her energy draining, her tensions increasing; many blue-collar workers whose jobs require vigorous activity for parts of the body; weekend athletes who think that tennis is an adequate conditioning program.

When you have a desire for good health, it's unfortunate that the problem is a lack of reliable information on nutrition and exercise because if you glance at the triangle again, you see that it takes very little effort to move upward into the basic fitness level.

Basic Fitness, Area B. Basic fitness, or good health, is what preventive medicine is all about, and its importance is easily explained. Because there is no cure for the major diseases, basic fitness is the only protection against such maladies as cancer, stroke, and heart disease. Furthermore, it's estimated that as much as 90 percent of all illness is caused by poor nutrition, lack of proper exercise, and habits such as smoking and excessive drinking —all factors which doctors don't control. Our only protection is good health. To paraphrase Vince Lombardi:

FITNESS ISN'T EVERYTHING. IT'S THE ONLY THING.

The payoff is dramatic for the person who moves into the basic fitness level. A six-year California study of 7,000 adults found that those with good health factors, including attention to nutrition and exercise, moderate drinking, and the elimination of smoking, were at the upper level of good health. In the age range of 55 to 64 these people had the health status of 25- to 34-year olds who gave little or no attention to health factors. The middle-aged in good health were up to "30 years younger" than others in their generation. But younger people in their twenties and thirties who neglected their health were living in their middle years.

The lower part of B in the triangle would be the beginning level of basic conditioning; the top would be the maintenance level to ensure enough fitness to get through every day in good health, eliminating chronic complaints of stress and aches and improving stamina to a degree that gets one through a day's work with enough energy left over for social activities and what the individual defines as desirable sexual activity.

Sex is not usually the most demanding activity in daily living, but we continue to hear about the too tired/headache syndrome as a common problem in sexual dysfunction. To be satisfactory rather than perfunctory, sex requires stamina, both mental and sensual, and muscular function, including flexibility and strength, but to a much lesser degree than most athletic activity.* However, just as in any other context, how much fitness depends on the individual.

Recent reports tell us that well-conditioned athletes, including those in the weekend category, have sex frequently (daily, they say) and that each period lasts a full hour, compared to a general average of twelve times a month with an average period of twenty minutes. The reports on the athlete's sex life aren't scientific. We don't know if both partners are in excellent condition or one is passive. Furthermore, we don't know if endurance has anything to do with the quality of sex, although there is a cult of long-distance runners who subscribe to the overall philosophy that the longer, the better.

Still, there is universal agreement in the medical profession that fitness is a major factor in the enjoyment of sex. Athletic fitness

---

* Cardiologist Campbell Moses, formerly medical director of the American Heart Association, observes that sexual activity is anaerobic about "equal to a sprint up two flights of stairs." The pulse may rise as high as 150 heartbeats per minute, but 120 is average at the point of orgasm. Dr. Moses recommends non-calisthenic warm-up and cool-off periods. (For the record, the authors wish to disassociate themselves from the implication that sex is an athletic performance.)

may not make a good lover, but it's doubtful that you can be one without good health. However, the presumption that good health automatically turns a person into a spectacular bed partner is just as false as the assumption that good health is all that's necessary to get into weekend sports activity.

The essential good feeling that comes with basic fitness is misleading because it is fitness for a life-style that is sedentary. As a result, those who maintain themselves in the basic fitness/good health category suffer the majority of sport injuries when they get into weekend athletics. If they are lucky enough to avoid serious injury, they show up the next day at work or school complaining of sore muscles or tendons. On the subtle side, but devastating, is the loss of confidence in their game. They are losers because basic fitness doesn't prepare them to compete.

Athletic Fitness. The difference between basic and athletic fitness is again answered by putting the question "Fit for what?" Basic fitness is designed to maintain good health in a life context that is generally sedentary. The athlete, on the other hand, is concerned with a greater measure of vigor and body movement. The question becomes: "Fit for what level of sports activity?"

Area D gives you an idea of the effort and work required of scheduled athletes—those who participate in scheduled competition, train at scheduled practices, and are supervised by coaches, trainers, and team doctors. Conditioning in this area is not worth the effort of the weekend athlete, even if the time is available. Businessmen will tell you that the money and effort required to reach the optimum in production and sales are not worth the cost. Beyond a certain point the return is too small related to the time, effort and dollars invested.

A similar principle is involved in the work of scheduled athletes. You get less for the effort as you near the optimum of fitness, although it is this small difference that is critical at the world-class level, where a fraction of a second separates the winner from the loser. The world-class athlete is a highly dedicated and disciplined person who in effect pays "top price" for optimum fitness. It's not necessary for the weekender even if the weekender has the available time. The extra time would be better spent in developing skills for another sport.

What may appear contradictory in Area D is placing the college athlete over the professional. The pro is more skilled but will sustain more injuries than the college competitor, and that's because the college athlete is in better condition. Throughout the school year, about ten months, the coach and trainers supervise conditioning, and during the vacation period it's common practice to arrange a summer job that will maintain conditioning. On the other hand, when the professional season is over, the coaching staff and players split to go home to hunt and fish. When a pro maintains conditioning off-season, it's a personal decision and personal planning that may not have the benefit of sports medicine specialists.

The difference in conditioning between the pro and weekender is a lot more substantial than the continuum triangle indicates, but from a lifetime perspective the weekender may be in a healthier position than the pro. For many professional athletes, retirement means the elimination of the "physical work." They don't have guidance in cutting back from intense to moderate workouts, 30 pounds of muscle becomes 30 pounds of fat,* and as a result, they go from lean and strong to flabby and pudgy. The lack of exercise and poor nutrition suddenly age the pros and make them susceptible to disease.

Here again we have the dichotomy mentality—scheduled athletes who believe that the choice is either a heavy conditioning schedule or nothing when conditioning at a weekend level is all that they need at retirement to maintain skills.

Summary

Returning to the diagram, "Physical Fitness Continuum Triangle," the following would be an estimate of effort needed to reach the various levels of fitness:

FITNESS LEVEL A: POOR FITNESS/HEALTH

—Little or no effort expended beyond that which is necessary for day-to-day existence in sedentary work.

* Muscle does not literally turn into fat. Without use/exercise, the muscle atrophies. If the athlete continues to consume calories at the same level, the muscle is replaced by fat in total body weight.

FITNESS LEVEL B: BASIC FITNESS

—May be obtained with as little as 15 to 30 minutes work 3 times a week.

—Intensity level is low.

—Most people need help in developing a program. The conditioning prescribed at Step 1, GAF level I, in this book would be appropriate. See Part II.

FITNESS LEVEL C: THE WEEKEND ATHLETE

—May be obtained with 35 to 50 minutes of work 3 times a week.

—Intensity level is moderate.

—Virtually all weekend athletes need help in developing this program, which is provided in this book in Part II, "GAF" and Part IV, "The Physical Edge."

FITNESS LEVEL D: SCHEDULED ATHLETES

—For vigorous sports, the amount of time required is substantial—3 hours or more daily throughout most of the year.

—For vigorous sports, the level of intensity is high to very high.

—Successful athletes at this level require the best in professional coaching.

The difference between weekend and scheduled athletic fitness is in the degree of conditioning. An athletic profile for weekenders and scheduled athletes includes the same components:

1. BODY COMPOSITION: the relative composition of lean body mass (muscle), body fat, bone, and other vital organs and parts. Determining a person's body composition gives you far better information about fitness and proficiency than either appearance or the body weight numbers you get off the bathroom scales. For example, a study on a college campus found that some young men who appeared to be slender actually had a higher percentage of body fat than the huskier members of the football squad.

There are three factors that determine body composition. One is managing calorie intake and output to prevent an accumulation of excess body fat. Another is maintaining muscle tissue at a level that will permit you to participate in work, social, and athletic activities. The third factor is genetics, but this is of consequence only for the professional or world-class competitor. For example, Olympic champion Frank Shorter is reported to have only 2 or 3 percent body fat. It would be virtually impossible for most weekend athletes to get that low without several generations of genetic engineering.

2. STRENGTH: the amount of force that a muscle or muscle group can exert. For example, to be able to do one push-up tells you that you have enough strength in your arms and shoulder girdle to lift two-thirds of your body weight off the floor.

3. MUSCULAR ENDURANCE: the ability of a muscle or muscle groups to exert external force repetitively.

4. FLEXIBILITY: the ability to move through the full range of motion of a particular joint or combination of joints.

5. AGILITY: the ability to change direction rapidly.

6. COORDINATION: the ability to combine the use of various parts of the body to produce efficient patterned movements.

7. REACTION TIME: in the context of sports it is the time required to initiate a movement of various body parts after the reception of a visual or auditory stimulus.

8. CARDIORESPIRATORY ENDURANCE: the ability of the circulatory and respiratory systems to supply nutrients and oxygen in adequate amounts during sustained physical activity.

All the above are dependent on exercise physiology, although nutrition is also a major factor in body composition.

Chapter 7

The Athletic Profile—A Very Informative Chapter

The Fitness Components

1. Agility	4. Cardiorespiratory	7. Muscular Strength
2. Body	Endurance	8. Nutrition
Composition	5. Flexibility	9. Reaction Time
3. Coordination	6. Muscular	
	Endurance	

It's one thing to list the components of athletic fitness and another to know how to develop them. The implication that most athletes, coaches, and trainers know what they are doing should be qualified. Most of the sophistication is at the world-class and college level. At the professional, high school, and weekend level of sports, the existing conditions may be a little hairy. As an illustration let's look at a composite, but not fictional, football team.

Good ole coach tells his team to avoid swimming during summer pretraining to keep muscles from going soft.

The idea that swimming is a kind of sissy sport continues to prevail, although today's competitive swimmers frequently use weight training to increase strength. Swimming itself contributes to muscular endurance and flexibility and, when performed at the proper level, can improve the cardiorespiratory system just as running does. Swimming is not necessary in pretraining, but it is more likely to be an asset than a handicap.

Curiously, a very competitive weekend swimmer told us that she doesn't run when she's in training because she's afraid that running will interfere with her swimming muscles, and that's another myth.

66

Remember, pentathlon competitors must run, swim, ride, fence, and shoot. And each sport requires different motor skills.

Good ole coach encourages his players to put on weight to become big and strong.

In fact, it is not bigness that is a factor in measuring strength, but body composition—the ratio of body fat to lean body mass. When a man's body fat edges over 13 to 15 percent and a woman's over 18 to 20 percent, cardiorespiratory and muscular endurance falls off. As a result, you have a player whose tongue begins to hang out before the game is over. Furthermore, overall motor fitness suffers, meaning poor performance—a loss of agility, speed, and power.

It is a common error to equate a beefy athlete with power when, in truth, lean means power. Although we associate brute strength with American football, a study of the best performers on a professional team found that the ideal amount of body fat should be at 8 percent for defensive and offensive backs and at 15 percent for linebackers, offensive linemen, and tight ends. And that is lean.

Power improvement can be explained mathematically. For example, when Chuck Ramsey, one of the nation's best punters, put on weight, his record fell off so badly that he was cut from the squad. When Ramsey dropped 20 pounds, he returned to professional play to record an impresive 45.1 average. Now for the arithmetic. Suppose Ramsey's leg thrust is 1000 pounds and he weighs 205. You have a ratio of 1,000 to 205 or 4.8 to 1. When his weight drops to 185, the ratio is about 5.4 to 1, a power increase of about 11 percent as a result of fat loss.

There are some other athletes who are also smart enough to recognize the effect of overfat on performance. Professional hockey player Brent Hughes testified in court, "If I'm ten to fifteen pounds overweight, I can't perform. I'm fighting for my job."

All this information is important to the weekend athlete because the average American man has about 25 percent body fat and the average woman over 30 percent—enough to handicap performance seriously.

Very few weekend athletes have the facilities available to determine body composition. Therefore, we should consider overweight to be overfat. Virtually all of us, including those who do not look fat in street clothes, would gain measurable benefits in performance with a loss of 5 to 25 pounds in total body weight. This would directly lower body fat percentage.

Ole coach runs the team up and down stadium steps to develop leg strength.

Running up steps helps strengthen the quadriceps (see diagram on page 206), but running down is likely to result in strain and injury to feet and knees. The reason: Biomechanical analysis finds that running down steps or downhill exerts four times the body weight on feet.

One of ole coach's favorite conditions is running the team in wind sprints to develop cardiorespiratory endurance and speed.

"Wind sprints" is a misnomer because the sprint is an anaerobic exercise that develops neither wind nor speed, and there's a simple explanation for this. When an activity is very demanding, such as a sprint, there is no time for the muscles to draw oxygen from the bloodstream to produce energy. Instead, the muscles draw energy from nonoxidative sources, mainly the glycogen stored in the muscle tissue.

The muscles work fine until the store of glycogen is expended—usually after 8 to 10 short sprints or about 2 minutes of strenuous and continuous sprinting. When the glycogen stored in the muscles is depleted, the muscles stop contracting, and the runner drops from exhaustion. During this brief, vital period of anaerobic activity the cardiorespiratory system has been shut out by the muscles.* On the other hand, aerobic exercises develop cardiorespiratory endurance because the activity is moderate rather than strenuous and of longer duration, usually more than 5 minutes.

When muscles are used over a long period of time, the blood delivers oxygen to the muscles to oxidate energy from nutrients in the bloodstream and the tissues. This kind of exercise gives the cardiorespiratory system a workout, thereby increasing its efficiency—the heart delivers more blood per stroke, the respiratory muscles are strengthened, the hemoglobin count increases, and the blood vessels expand and become more flexible. As a result of this conditioning,

---

* For the record, wind sprints neither correct biomechanical problems to increase speed nor increase strength to improve quickness.

muscles retain maximum strength longer when it comes time to compete.

One of the keys to developing cardiorespiratory endurance is to run *strong and relaxed* for long periods, preferably 20 minutes or more but not less than 10 minutes. If you are either a football player or weekender who plays tennis, handball, or any other sport that requires both quickness and cardiorespiratory endurance, you would begin training by running *relaxed* for distances of from 880 yards/.792 kilometer to 1 mile/1.6 kilometer at least 3 times a week for about 8 weeks. This should be not a jog, but more a striding, loose-styled run.

Each week run a little faster or a little farther. During the last three or four weeks, in addition to the loose-styled run of a mile or more, begin running up hills or stadium steps in striding short runs of 40 or 50 yards or steps, gradually increasing the number of short runs or steps. The uphill run helps develop leg strength and thus increases quickness. Plan the uphill runs at the end of the workout so that you can walk back down as a cooling-off exercise.

After 8 weeks you may begin to include interval training runs. The pace, length, and frequency of the runs depend upon the position the player fills, whether he is a lineman or a back, on the defensive or offensive team. For the weekend athlete, this will be prescribed by individual sports in Part IV.

Good ole coach forbids drinking water during workouts, even during the very warm days of August and early September.

He may believe that giving fluids to an athlete is as dangerous as pouring ice water into a hot glass. Or he may believe, as did a high school coach near West Point, that restricting fluids during practice "toughens" up the team.

Today we know that fluids are recommended during strenuous workouts and that abstinence occasionally results in sudden death. Working on a hot day can quickly dehydrate anyone no matter how well conditioned the person may be. Even in the relative cool of a gymnasium a vigorous handball game can cost a player 3 to 5 pounds of fluid in an hour.

The error of the coach is in not understanding that virtually every organ in the body is dependent on an adequate supply of fluid to function—fluid is in the muscles, fluid lubricates the joints, and fluid is essential to maintain the flow of oxygen in the body. During physical activity the body is totally dependent on fluid to carry off excessive internal heat.

The well-publicized collapse of President Jimmy Carter during a run was caused by heat exhaustion according to his physician. The usual cause of heat exhaustion is insufficient fluids to dissipate internal body heat. A step up, and worse, is heat stroke, which is often fatal. This whole matter can be summarized by remembering that the body is a "water-cooled engine." You have to keep the radiator full.

On the day of the game the team goes on a heavy diet of protein, a breakfast that may include eggs and bacon and sausage, and, at midday, a big steak.

Our Greek friend Milo would have savored this menu. Milo was known to backpack a heifer into the arena, kill it with one blow from his fist, and then eat the whole thing. Perhaps inspired by Milo, ancient Greek trainers recommended meat diets to athletes, especially wrestlers and boxers, so the myth about meat began and prevailed. It was more than 2,000 years before research taught us that carbohydrates, not protein, are preferred by the brain and muscles as a source of energy.

We have learned more about human nutrition in the twentieth century than in the whole history of man, and this began with the introduction of the biological analysis of foods by Verner McCollum at the University of Wisconsin early in the century. Today we know that a high-protein diet is a poor way to prepare for a game or any other activity.

Protein is not the best source of energy, but primarily a substance that builds and repairs body tissue. Only excesses of protein turn into fat and subsequently into calories for energy, and that takes a long time. Usually the pregame steak is still in the digestive tract of the athlete when the band and baton twirlers come marching on the field during half time.

Protein has become an obsession with many who want to exert maximum physical and sexual power, but modern research finds that the athlete, pound for pound, requires no more protein than anyone else. Virtually all Americans get more than enough protein and far too much dietary fat, as indicated in research:

Calorie Intake of	Actual	Recommended
Fat	45%	22%
Protein	14%	12%
Carbohydrates	41%	66%

The recommended carbohydrate increase is not an invitation to fill up on the simple sugar carbohydrates, but a strong recommendation to move into the complex carbohydrates which we know as starches, including the cereals, legumes, and tubers such as the potato. These foods are excellent sources of energy which the body stores as glycogen (and which the body cannot make from either fat or protein). In addition, these starches contribute vitamins, minerals, fiber, and protein.

The pregame meal should contain only a little protein and fat because both these nutrients take longer to digest than carbohydrates. Furthermore, meats and eggs are acid-forming and thus may contribute to acidosis during competition. For these and other reasons, the pregame meal should be mainly complex carbohydrates with a total energy intake of no more than 750 calories. The meal should be scheduled at least four hours before competition, but you can drink fluids right up to game time, and you may continue to sip fluids during the game.

Another pregame tradition of good ole coach is warming up the team with push-ups, sit-ups, and other muscle builders.

This is an exercise in wishful thinking because the pregame period is a little late to begin strengthening the team. The pregame period is the time for flexibility exercises to prepare muscles for action. Although more and more people know this, many don't know that there are two types of flexibility—static and dynamic. Static flexibility refers to the range of movement of a particular joint, while dynamic flexibility refers to the ease with which a joint moves through its range of motion during activity.

Some coaches don't know about dynamic flexibility, and you will see pictures of professional teams warming up with exercises that may be more appropriate to deep meditation. Furthermore, some coaches don't understand that although flexibility is a major component in promoting mobility and preventing injury, it is different from other components. For example, we know that being a little faster, stronger, and quicker is better and improves athletic performance. However, with flexibility enough is enough, and too much is as much of a risk as too little.

Inflexibility is a common problem, but it can just as easily be the curse of both the sedentary or the active person. For example, sitting much of the day shortens the hamstring muscle, so when we suddenly reach over to pick up a ball or pencil, we hurt our backs, but actually it is the hamstring as well as the back muscle that is strained. Or a woman who constantly wears high heels shortens her Achilles tendon, so when she puts on sneakers or running shoes, the tendon is wrenched.

The weekend athlete or pro suffers the same problems when he takes to muscle-strengthening exercises that aren't programmed to use the full range of movement.

In recent years there has been extensive research in muscle flexibility, including original studies at West Point. Happily for the weekender, flexibility is the least demanding of any conditioning exercises and requires only a few minutes. This book will deal mainly with dynamic flexibility, which is the athlete's concern.

And Now the Truth About Muscle Builders

If you're old enough to remember George Atlas ads, then you remember the bully kicked sand in the skinny guy's face and walked off with all the pretty girls until the skinny guy bought the muscle-building equipment, built up his physique, and powed the bully. That appeared to be the only reason to pump iron because we had mechanical forks, tractors, and other kinds of machinery to lift, push, and move heavy material, thus doing away with the need for strong men.

Since those distant days man has come to believe that body building is a sign of undernourished ego or flagrant machismo, so muscle building has fallen into disrepute. There are exceptions—we may appreciate the football player who can muscle through the defense to nail the ballcarrier, but that admiration is seasonal.

What we continue to admire is agility, coordination, good reflexes, flexibility, power, and speed—qualities that make a good tennis player, golfer, dancer, skier, swimmer, and that's the catch. All these qualities are dependent on strengthening muscles. That's why you hear of pretty little swimmers and slim pitchers getting into muscle-developing programs. They are not into the body beautiful syndrome. The little girl wants to increase her speed in the pool, and the pitcher wants to get his ball speed over 90 miles an hour. Sports research has taught us that virtually any athlete, from the weekender to the Olympic gold medal winner, will improve performance with strength training.

Many of us have poor understanding of the function of muscles. We continue to be locked into the cultural implication that strong is always bulky and mountainous. We don't perceive that the slender teenage girl aced her way into Wimbledon with muscle. We even lose sight of the fact that if it weren't for muscles, we couldn't sit, pick up a fork, or switch on the car ignition.

We forget lessons in elementary anatomy, that bones really aren't much more than tent poles. Take away the ropes, and the poles fall down, the tent collapses. Similarly, if muscles aren't doing minimal work, the body will collapse when you try to stand. It's not the fever or virus that weakened you. Your weakness is muscular. You must gradually strengthen your muscles again.

You maintain muscular strength to walk around by walking around every day. If you swim forty-five minutes every day, you will maintain enough strength to swim forty-five minutes a day. You've set a limit to your mobility and performance. However, if you want to swim competitively or compete in any sport, then your muscles require an extra degree of conditioning to develop power and speed, agility and endurance, coordination and good reaction time.

Power and Speed, Every Competitor's Desire

Power, the primary advantage in almost any sport, is the result of strength and speed. Strength by itself increases the impact made on a ball, but it also increases speed of movement in arms and legs, and this, too, increases the force at impact. The product of strength and speed is a substantial increase in power. That explains why muscle-building exercises are essential to the youngster who wants to develop a "powerful swimming stroke," the big-league pitcher who wants to power in his fast ball, and the weekender who wants a powerful drive or serve.

Speed, as we commonly use the word, meaning to run fast on a field or track or to move fast on a court, is dependent on leg and lower-torso strength. Speed may be improved substantially, the limiting factor being genetics—the fast- and slow-twitch muscles noted earlier. Although strength and endurance can be improved by 50 percent or more (at West Point, we've increased the overall strength of some men and women by 100 percent), an increase of running speed of as much as 15 percent is unusual.

For the weekend athlete who isn't involved in split-second competition, a reasonable goal is working to get back most of the speed of youth. Some track coaches have used running up steep hills to strengthen muscles and thus increase speed. At West Point we've been successful in increasing running speed by strengthening muscles of the low back, hips, and legs through isotonic and isokinetic training, and these techniques will be passed along to you in Part II, "GAF", and Part IV, "The Physical Edge."

RT, Coordination, and Agility

Another component, RT (reaction time), can also be improved by increasing strength. Neurologically RT depends on the length of the neural pathway from the receptor organ, such as the eye or ear, to the limb muscle, including the time it takes the brain to process the information and get the neural signals on the way. Overall RT is a combination of several factors, including strength, neurological response, and speed of movement. Another factor is anticipation. With experience, athletes develop the ability to anticipate what an opponent will do next and thus begin moving before the stimulus is made available to the brain.

In lab studies, men have demonstrated slightly better RT than women, enough to give a man a competitive edge. RT for both men and women reaches its peak between the ages of 20 and 30, then falls off as they get older. However, the decrease is very gradual, virtually imperceptible for the active person. In fact, maintaining activity and conditioning slows the aging process in general and at the same time helps retain good RT.

Agility and *coordination* are two components that may be inter-defined. Exercise physiologists define agility as the ability to change direction rapidly, coordination as the ability to move with smooth, balanced, and fluid motions. Both are dependent on muscular strength, muscular endurance, and flexibility, but agility and coordination are then specifically developed by practice of the movements of a specific sport or activity such as a dance.

For example, a handball player must develop the necessary hand-eye coordination to hit the ball just as the soccer player requires foot-eye coordination. The player begins by concentrating on the ball, what is called the sensory set, and this is followed by the motor set, moving into position to intercept the ball and return it. During the learning period the player thinks through the movement, and this is called conscious control. As skill improves, the movement occurs automatically through conditioned or learned reflexes. Agility and coordination are most efficiently developed when prescribed for specific sports. How you go about this is explained in full in Part IV, "The Physical Edge."

All the fitness components, with the exception of nutrition, depend on muscular conditioning as either the major or supporting factor. Modern sports medicine not only provides the most efficient methods but also guarantees that although you may never be as strong as a Greek wrestler or a Dallas Cowboy, you are likely to be in better all-around muscular condition than the Milos of the past and present.

Chapter 8

Muscle Conditioning—Myth, Matter, and Good-bye, Milo

When Milo of Crotona swaggered into the coliseum locker room with a live cow slung over his shoulders, some of the other athletes thought he was just an ornery farm boy. Others figured that he was trying to psych his opponents.

One gladiator cracked, "It looks as if Milo brought his lunch."

No joke. It was his lunch, but the farm boy was also demonstrating an understanding of muscle conditioning that in modern times is known as the principle of progressive conditioning.

According to myth, Milo carried a heifer over his shoulders from its day of birth. From day to day the heifer (resistance) grew heavier. In turn, Milo's muscles, in adapting to the ever-increasing overload, grew stronger. This roughly illustrates the modern principle of progressive conditioning. However, for all of Milo's ingenuity and prowess, if he had tried to go up for a rebound, drive a golf ball, or return a lob, he would likely have tied himself into knots.

There are many modern Milos who can't participate in more than one sport at a time because they aren't taking advantage of the state of art in exercise physiology. If a program is properly designed, you can develop symmetrical and full-motion strength with no risk of becoming muscle-bound. That disposes of one myth, but there are others that continue to handicap many people.

Myth: From age 40 on muscles begin to atrophy rapidly.

Not true. Men and women are competing in tennis, golf, swim meets, and other sport events through their seventies and into their eighties. If you maintain muscle conditioning at a moderate level, you can just about go on forever. When not used, muscles atrophy.

Myth: Women's muscles are not capable of performing the hard work demanded in most sports.

False, but West Point doesn't take the irresponsible position that women can participate in any game with men. The Academy believes that women would suffer a great amount of injury if permitted to compete with men in football, lacrosse, wrestling, and most other contact sports because men are more powerful. Men outweigh, outmuscle, and outsize women, thus giving men an unfair physical advantage. However, West Point women are otherwise free to compete with men in any other sport, academically, or in any other way they wish.

Myth: Women develop bulky muscles when they get into weight-training programs.

West Point has documented studies proving that virtually all women and some men can take over 100 percent gains in strength without muscle hypertrophy, although most men do show an increase in muscle size. It's hypothesized that the predominantly male sex hormone testosterone accounts for male hypertrophy and that the low level of testosterone in women makes the occurrence of bulky muscles virtually impossible.

Myth: Women cannot perform at a competitive level in most American games.

False. Although most women don't have the opportunity to learn sport skills as youngsters, at West Point we are having a significant measure of success in improving the athletic performance of women cadets, and much of this success is a result of strength increases in their hands, arms, and shoulders.

When women enter the Academy, they are likely to have difficulty handling a basketball, directing a tennis ball, or moving strongly through water. In the beginning plebe women let many passes slip through their hands, and they have difficulty making the long pass or the fast break or catching the ball at the end of the fast break. But with the increase of upper-torso and arm and wrist strength, women become much more adept at handling a ball, striking a ball, and moving better in water sports. The weekend athlete, man or woman, is guaranteed similar improvement in sport performance, and the sedentary person, who is among the mass of people entering recreational sports for the first time, has everything to gain from this program.

Muscular conditioning of the lower torso and legs is as important in promoting mobility as it is in preventing injury to feet, knees, and hips. Here again, contemporary society has the advantage of the current research in sports medicine. Briefly we'd like to review some of the principles and theories that confuse the public.

The Buzz Words and the Reality

Research has taught us that there are three procedures in strength development—isometric, isotonic and isokinetic. Unfortunately these have become buzz words for many of us. We know the words but don't understand how they relate to the weekend athlete.

Isometric (static) procedures are not new but made a big come-back in the 1950's as a result of studies made by Mueller and Hettinger in Germany. They claimed remarkable strength gains with isometric conditioning. Recent research refutes some of their findings and has discovered other drawbacks and limitations in isometrics.

Isometric conditioning is simply pitting one's muscles against an unmovable object, such as a wall. During the effort the muscles remain static, meaning there is no change in muscle length. Only the muscle fibers contract. If you apply maximum effort during an isometric exercise, maximum fiber fatigue follows. The body then responds by rebuilding the muscle fiber to a stronger level.

Generally the best results from isometrics are obtained by holding maximum contractions for 6 seconds, followed by a 6-second rest period with 5 to 10 repetitions every day. The major fault in isometrics is the failure to put muscles through the full range of motion.

Isometric contraction develops strength only at a single point in the range of motion. A contraction at 90 degrees with your hands pushing against walls does little to develop strength at 40 or 135 degrees. So now you have the awkward and complicated task of performing contractions at different angles in order to develop strength through the full range of motion. Furthermore, isometrics interferes with blood circulation. When the muscles are static, the contraction of muscle fibers alone constricts the blood vessels. This may raise blood pressure and pose a risk to a person with hypertension. On the other hand, during isotonic and isokinetic conditioning, the whole muscle contracts, and as a result, there is no interference with blood circulation. This is also a plus in conditioning because blood circulation must be involved in improving muscular endurance.

Both *isotonics* and *isokinetics* involve the movement of joints and muscles coupled with the resistant. The classic comparison of isometrics with isotonics can be found in the story of Samson. When Delilah cut Samson's hair, robbing him of his strength, Samson couldn't budge the pillars in the temple. His muscles strained without contracting. This was isometric. When his hair grew back and he had the strength to move the pillars, he was performing a modified isotonic exercise.*

In isotonic movements the weight of resistance is constant throughout the full range of motion. A 100-pound barbell remains 100 pounds through the entire lift. However, because of the construction of the arm and elbow, the amount of weight that can be lifted depends on the position of the arm.

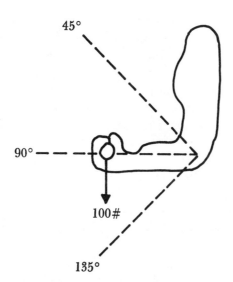

---

* Samson was a sensuous handsome man and Delilah, a sensuous beautiful woman. The adult interpretation of their story concludes that their interest was conjugal rather than tonsorial, and since that time the myth has prevailed that sexual activity weakens an athlete. Although research is limited, most authorities agree that normal sexual activity seldom interferes with athletic performance. Manager Casey Stengel once observed that it wasn't sex that tired out his ballplayers so much as the long hours spent in its pursuit.

The arm supports maximum weight at the 90-degree angle. If the maximum weight that you are able to support at 90 degrees is 100 pounds, then at 45 degrees you would be able to support only 65 pounds, and at 135 degrees, only 45 pounds, to work through the full range of motion.

Now, however, new variable resistance equipment has been developed to overcome this problem. This equipment maintains the intensity of resistance no matter what the angle of the arm. The name given this conditioning is isokinetics. (For more detail on isokinetic equipment, see "Weight Lifting," page 309.)

The major problem in isokinetic conditioning is that most of us, including some professional athletes, lack time, equipment, and proper supervision. Therefore, of the three strength-development procedures, isotonics is the most practical and important to the weekend athlete.

Traditionally isotonics has involved the use of free weights as resistance, including barbells, dumbbells, and wall pulleys. In calisthenics, body weight is the resistance and is very effective as we realize in doing push-ups, pull-ups, and even sit-ups. In the past isotonic training has been haphazard and seldom, if ever, used efficiently. Today exercise physiology makes it possible to prescribe specific exercises for specific sports and thereby develop two important components—muscular strength and muscular endurance.

Finally, the Scientific Answer: When More/Less Is Better

The relationship between muscular strength and muscular endurance was first recognized by T. L. DeLorme in the mid-1940's. DeLorme found that strength is developed by lifting heavy weights for a few repetitions, but muscular endurance requires many repetitions of lifting light weights. DeLorme's Principle is diagrammed on the opposite page.

The ratio between weights and repetitions is relative, differing for each person. For example, *light weight/high repetitions* refers to the weight that a person can move for 20 or more repetitions. However, the weight must be heavy enough that somewhere close to 20 repetitions the muscles become fatigued. The heavy weight in *heavy weight/low repetitions* would be an object that can be moved

DeLORME'S PRINCIPLE

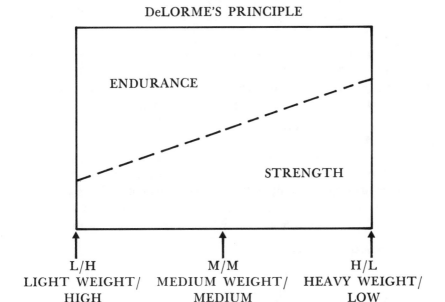

three or four times. The interpretation of the diagram is easy enough:

> L/H: Light weights and high number of repetitions build endurance and a little strength.
>
> M/M: Medium weights and medium number of repetitions develop strength and endurance about equally.
>
> H/L: Heavy weights and a low number of repetitions mainly develop strength and some muscular endurance.

Suppose your upper-torso strength is under par. You can do two or three push-ups off the floor. You would do three push-ups daily to build strength, and then you would do about twenty push-ups off the wall to build up muscular endurance. Or you might go the middle route, pushing off a bed with your feet on the floor.

DeLorme's Principle applies whether you are using body weight or weight-training equipment. In this book we will use body weight so that conditioning may be done at home, at your convenience, and at no expense.

Basic Principles for Strength and Endurance Improvement

Sports medicine has brought not only understanding to athletic fitness but also order in planning conditioning programs. The guides are based on the following five principles which you may care to glance at to understand the West Point program:

PRINCIPLE I: OVERLOAD

To increase muscular strength and endurance, the muscles must be worked a little harder than normal. For example, if you can do three push-ups comfortably, then you exert yourself above the comfort range to do four or five. If you can't do a single push-up, then you begin by pushing off a wall or by doing negative push-ups.

PRINCIPLE II: PROGRESSION

The overload, or resistance, must be increased gradually in order to increase either strength or endurance.

PRINCIPLE III: USE/DISUSE

The fundamental principle of physical conditioning stems from the knowledge that the healthy body thrives on use. Conversely, if the body is not used, deterioration sets in. The lack of body use has been identified as the cause of a broad range of health problems— from low-back pain to heart disease and emotional instability.

For the active weekend athlete, the principle of Use/Disuse translates into maintenance. Once an individual chooses and reaches a level of fitness appropriate to her/his life-style, it must be maintained. In this book we begin by establishing a readiness level that we call General Athletic Fitness.

PRINCIPLE IV: SPECIFICITY

Although a good program is concerned with all the components of fitness, the level of conditioning for the different components depends on the weekender's favorite game, the specific biomechanical demands of a specific sport.

PRINCIPLE V: INDIVIDUAL DIFFERENCES

Levels of athletic fitness not only depend on the specific sport but must also include age, health, and level of competition. At the weekend level we are concerned with a degree of readiness that ensures maximum performance on the job and in your favorite game. Since most people today are engaged in sedentary work, this usually means bringing the individual's endurance and strength up to the level required by the specific sport.

The above principles should be remembered if and when you decide to adapt any conditioning program for special needs, and perhaps by now you have read as much as you want to know about the state of the art. This may also be the time to say good-bye to Milo of Crotona, who first instructed us in overload and progression but then left us with mistaken ideas on nutrition and brute strength that unfortunately dominated sports for some 2,500 years.

There was poetic justice in Milo's exit, an environmental reckoning in his death. This came about when Milo attempted to split a tree with a karate chop. His hand became wedged in the tree trunk, and Milo was trapped. That evening he was recycled by a pack of wolves.

Except for an occasional weight lifter such as Vasily Alexeyev, there are few great athletes who resemble Milo. The best professional football players may be big, but they are fairly well balanced in muscular development and body composition. Even the new breed of wrestlers are lean.

Farewell, Milo.

PART II

General Athletic Fitness:
The Winner's Circuit

Your Power Base

Chapter 9

GAF—General Athletic Fitness— What and How Much?

The information in this part of the book is guaranteed to improve your performance within two or three weeks. We make that statement because we worry that the competitive weekender will turn ahead to specific conditioning for a favorite sport. If you bypass this section, you will be cheated of basic power and flexibility, two factors that not only establish a sound competitive edge but also prevent strain, pain, and injury.

What Is GAF?

Earlier in the book basic fitness was defined as being sufficiently fit to accomplish each day's work and social activities with a little in reserve to meet an unexpected emergency. The components of basic fitness are health-related and include cardiorespiratory endurance, muscle strength, muscular endurance, flexibility, and body composition. The healthy organism should be maintained at the basic fitness level to remain stable. The absence of basic fitness is almost certain to bring on poor health and illness.

Although some sports, such as bowling and golf can be played at a noncompetitive level within the basic fitness zone, we must go a step farther in our conditioning for vigorous sports if we want to win. To do this, we must improve the components of basic fitness as well as those components that develop athletic skills. The athletic components are agility, balance, coordination, reaction time, and speed.* A schematic sketch of this concept looks something like this:

---

* Power is not noted in this context as an athletic skill because it is a combination of two other components—strength and speed.

WHAT IS GENERAL ATHLETIC FITNESS?

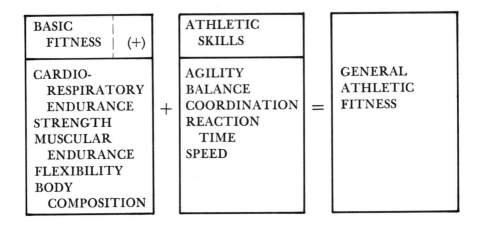

How Much GAF?

Logically, you may ask how much of each of these components is required to reach a satisfactory level of General Athletic Fitness.

If you ask the average coach how much conditioning a scheduled athlete requires in each of these components, the answer will be "as much as possible." In fact, the answer is not that simple, especially for the weekender. We all are different, and we all start out with different styles of play, physiques, and psychological attitudes that result in our using the components differently.

A sophisticated coach would begin by testing an athlete in the various athletic skills. If the athlete scores low on speed, the coach may emphasize interval running. You can do this for yourself when you get into the specific requirements of each sport to determine what conditioning you should emphasize.

The GAF conditioning program presented in this part of the book will help the weekender develop all components in the limited time available to a person fully occupied with a profession. The program is important to all weekend athletes who are participating in vigorous sports and those who want to develop a competitive edge in any sport.

The conditioning program is divided into three levels with three progressive steps within each level. You can choose the level that is most suitable to your style of play or favorite sport, and we provide a table (page 93) to guide you.

When Do You Use General Athletic Fitness?

The GAF program may be used at the lowest level to maintain a good state of basic fitness, but it is primarily designed for pre-season and in-season conditioning for the weekend athlete. If a seasonal sport is approaching, check the table (page 93) to see the level of conditioning required, and then, four to six weeks before the start of the season, begin to work yourself up to the appropriate level.

If you are in poor physical condition, start at GAF Level I; average condition, Level I or II; good condition, at any level you choose. However, Level III may be more difficult than you expect. Whatever level you choose, begin with the lowest progression step. Plan to stay with each step at least two weeks.

If you are already in-season, begin to work with the program on the days that you are not playing. You may be assured that you will see an improvement in your game and enjoy an absence of the normal aches that you have been putting up with. When you are in shape to sharpen your game, then refer to SAF—Specific Athletic Fitness (see Part IV).

GAF should be regarded with the same importance that you place on the solid foundation of a high-rise building. It supports your skills. The most vivid proof of this is the experience of our top athletes.

How Important Is GAF?

For the weekend athlete, General Athletic Fitness is more important than specific conditioning. We have proved this in studies of scores of men and women at West Point. Professional athletes have only recently learned to use GAF conditioning to salvage their careers and reduce their losses.

For example, when the world's best professional tennis players showed up for a world championship tennis final, seven of the eight stars (Bjorn Borg was the exception) brought with them traces of ailments that ranged from ankle and knee injuries to sprained wrists, tennis elbows, and bad backs. Two of the big names, and there's no need to embarrass them, admitted that they had used pain-killer drugs for muscle inflammation before discovering that the cure was in the muscular conditioning described in this part of the book.

The devastating effect that the lack of GAF can have on winning can be found on the sports page. Occasionally a coach can be embarrassingly ingenuous. Again, without using names, here is a typical example lifted off a sports page, describing a national basketball tournament. The nameless team was nine points ahead in the second half when, as the sportswriter noted, the team "went flat."

After the game the coach said, "We had five more minutes to play, but it came to a clear-cut point where we were just too tired."

Fatigue has nothing to do with skills. GAF conditioning builds the endurance base that is so important in winning.

In the opinion of most experts the lack of GAF conditioning has been mainly responsible for the humiliating defeats that the National Hockey League All-Stars have suffered when competing with the Russians. In 1972, when the Russians overpowered the Americans, the NHL admitted that its players were out of condition because the game was played during the off-season. However, the 1979 match was played during the in-season. The Russians whitewashed the NHL with a final score of 6 to 0. There was no mystery about this. The Russians were spending as much time in off-ice conditioning as they were with their on-ice skill practice.

During the 1980 Winter Olympics at Lake Placid, when the American hockey team upset the Russians, everyone was astonished. The skills of the Russians were so superior that one commentator compared the upset to that of a Canadian college football team defeating the Pittsburgh Steelers. The Americans were constantly aggressive, never letting up for a second. The only explanation was the high level of muscular and cardiorespiratory endurance of the American team, a testimonial to their conditioning, their coach, Herb Brooks, and the value of high-level General Athletic Fitness.

The lack of GAF is most prevalent in professional sports. Furthermore, many pros rest during the off-season. When they report for preseason training, the emphasis is on skills. For example, baseball teams spend so little time in spring training before they begin to play exhibition games that they have no time for GAF conditioning. This is thought to be the reason that so many injuries are incurred.

In Chapter 6, the diagram on page 58 shows the college athlete enjoying a higher level of conditioning than the pro. That's not because the college player is academically smarter. The reason is simply that the college coach supervises a team's conditioning for nine to ten months during the academic year and then makes arrangements to continue the conditioning during summer vacation.

Today the message that any competitive team has to work at GAF conditioning throughout the year is finally getting through. During the off-season the basic components are maintained at a higher level than is required for basic fitness. This is known as building the conditioning base. The preseason period is then used as a transitional period from GAF to SAF. However, GAF must continue right through the playing season.

Sports research has given us a fact that is irrefutable. If muscular strength and endurance, flexibility, and cardiorespiratory endurance are not continually reinforced by conditioning, these qualities deteriorate. On the other hand, athletic skills do not deteriorate as rapidly. Their reinforcement normally comes from practice drills and games. Understanding this, sophisticated coaches now continue strength and cardiorespiratory training through the playing season. Other coaches continue to sharpen skills and technique and then become perplexed because the overall performance of the team falls off. By the end of the playing season the team is actually weaker than it was at the beginning.

Here is a schematic of how a program should work in sports that are in-season during the fall:

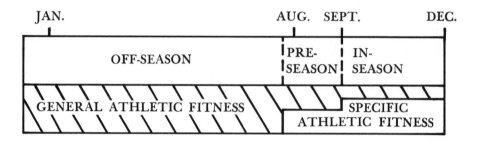

A GAF program for scheduled athletes should be designed to the needs of the sport. For example, a football team would require muscular strength and muscular endurance throughout the body. A soccer team would require muscular endurance and agility in the lower body and a much higher level of cardiorespiratory endurance. However, for the weekender, GAF conditioning can be more general and far less intensive. The weekender's GAF is based on two factors:

1. The degree of vigor demanded by the sport.
2. How vigorously and competitively he/she plays.

The table on the opposite page should be interpreted according to your needs. The weekender participating in light activity has no need to go beyond GAF Level I. The exception: If you golf or bowl at a very competitive level, you would be well served by conditioning at GAF Level II. On the other hand, if your sports activity requires that you condition at Level II but you occasionally get involved in a heavy sport such as basketball just for the fun of it, you would be foolish to push yourself into GAF Level III.

GAF Conditioning LEVEL I	GAF Conditioning LEVEL II	GAF Conditioning LEVEL III
LIGHT ACTIVITY SPORTS	MODERATE SPORTS ACTIVITY	HEAVY DUTY SPORTS
(or if you play a moderate activity sport just for the fun of it)	(or if you play a heavy activity sport just for the fun of it)	(or if you play a moderate activity sport in an all out, very competitive manner)

Archery
Bowling
Fishing
Golf
	Badminton
	Baseball/Softball
	Bicycling
	Downhill Skiing
	Fencing
	Horseback Riding
	Ice Skating
	Paddle Tennis—
	  Doubles
	Platform Tennis—
	  Doubles
	Roller Skating
	Scuba Diving
	Tennis—
	  Doubles
	Volleyball
		Basketball
		Cross-Country Skiing
		Judo
		Karate
		Handball
		Mountaineering
		Paddle Tennis—
		  Singles
		Platform Tennis—
		  Singles
		Racquetball/Paddle
		  Ball
		Running/Jogging
		Soccer
		Squash
		Swimming
		Tennis—Singles
		Touch Football
		Water Skiing
		Weight Lifting

Use your good sense in choosing the level that's best for you. Tune yourself according to your needs. As a general rule, however, if you want to play a strong game, you will improve your competitive edge by maintaining conditioning at a level higher than the sport calls for.

Before getting into the conditioning program, we want your

attention for several more pages to explain the importance of flexibility. We could give you a list of professional athletes the length of your arm who didn't discover flexibility until they had suffered injuries and muscular agony. We would prefer that you have the advantage of preventing the "crippling problems" of *in*flexibility.

Chapter 10

The Flexibility Advantage

By definition, flexibility is a measure of the range of motion available at a joint. Flexibility is determined by the shape of the bones and by the length of the ligaments and muscles that cross the joint. Range of flexibility varies by individuality and sex.

Generally, women are more flexible than men. It's a sucker bet if a woman brags that she can bend deeper from the hips than a man. Keeping her knees straight, she can likely touch the palms of her hands to the floor. A man in comparable condition does well to touch the floor with his fingertips. That's because a woman's legs are comparatively shorter, her torso is longer, and she has less muscle mass in the thighs (hamstrings) than a man.

Another unrealized fact is that too much flexibility is bad, impairs performance, and causes injuries. Excessive flexibility results in loose joints which lack stability, and this may lead to chronic injuries, especially in the knees and shoulder joints.

What we want for ourselves is a measure of flexibility that permits freedom of movement and, in turn, contributes to ease and economy of muscular effort, protects us against joint and muscular injury, and gives us a competitive edge.

To clear up some misunderstanding, here are some basic facts about flexibility:

• There is no one flexibility test that will measure a person's overall flexibility. It is specific to each joint of the body. Therefore, a greater degree of flexibility is desirable for specific joints depending on the demands of a specific sport. See Part IV, "The Physical Edge."

• Disuse is the cause of loss of flexibility in specific joints. The muscles have become shorter; the tendons, shorter. An example of disuse is a joint placed in a cast after an injury. When the cast comes off, we say, "The joint is stiff." Actually the muscles and tendons are as tight as they can be, and then, over a period of time, they have to be gradually stretched back to functional length. This is an extreme example of disuse. However, the sedentary person finds joints become inflexible because they are not used.

• Flexibility is affected by age not because of the aging process but primarily because many people become less active as they grow older. The very old may lose so much flexibility that they are afraid to walk for fear that they will fall. This is due solely to inactivity.

• Flexibility cannot be improved overnight or in a few days. Short muscles must be stretched gradually, over a period of weeks. On the other hand, a single flexibility exercise takes less than a minute a day.

• Flexibility must be maintained through brief daily exercises, but again, the time investment is minuscule, and stretching, like yawning, is in itself an exercise that relaxes the body.

• No one exercise will increase the flexibility of all muscles Different stretching exercises are required for the different muscle groups. The GAF stretching exercises in this book see to your overall flexibility. The SAF exercises see to the flexibility needs of a specific sport.

• Flexibility exercises fall into two categories: ballistic and static. The ballistic stretch is a bouncing or jerking motion that causes a stronger stretch. The static stretch is slow, sustained, and controlled; the muscle is lengthened and then held in the stretch for a brief time. The static stretch is preferable for the weekender because it eliminates the possibility of injury through overstretch.

• Being muscle-bound is simply a matter of muscle inflexibility. This occurs when an individual uses poor training procedures that result in muscles' being exercised unequally. For example, if the biceps muscles, the agonists, are strengthened more than the triceps muscles, the antagonists, the upper arm becomes muscle-bound. The stronger biceps overpower the triceps. You can see this in an athlete whose arms always bend somewhat instead of hanging straight down. Of course, not only the upper arm but any set of antagonistic pairs in the body may become muscle-bound.

The term "muscle-bound" is generally so misunderstood that the most authoritative dictionary, *Webster's Third New Inter-*

national Dictionary, states that the condition is caused by "excessive athletic activity." It is not a question of being excessive, but the kind of exercise.

We strongly recommend that you respect flexibility exercises. They are fundamental to performance and prevention of injury. Flexibility exercises included in GAF conditioning have been conscientiously designed for the weekender's needs.

On the following pages we will illustrate and give instructions for ten different flexibility/stretch exercises. These will be individually recommended for general athletic fitness and specific sports. You may wait and then learn only those that are called for, or you may choose to practice all ten to maintain an excellent level of flexibility.

ACHILLES STRETCH

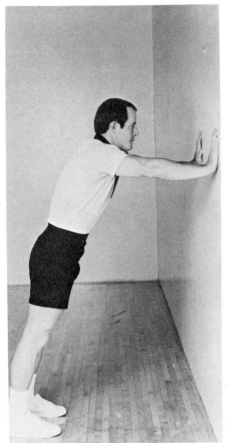

STARTING POSITION

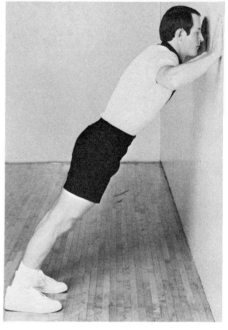

ACTION—
HOLD POSITION

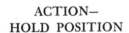

WARM-UP/COOL-DOWN/STRETCHING SERIES

INCREASING FLEXIBILITY TO HELP PREVENT INJURIES

1. *Achilles Stretch*

Purpose: To stretch the heel cords (Achilles tendons).

Starting Position: Stand about an arm's length from the wall— feet about four to five inches apart and parallel with toes perpendicular to the wall. Place hands on the wall at shoulder height and shoulder width apart.

Action: Bending the elbows, lean the body toward the wall while maintaining body alignment. Keep the heels on the floor, and continue to lean toward the wall until you feel a stretch in the calf of your legs; then hold for the prescribed count.

Cadence: Slow.

Progression: Start by holding for 15 seconds, and build up to 30 seconds. (Note: To count time accurately, use: "One-half and *one*, one-half and *two*, one-half and *three*," etc. up to a count of 15. Try timing yourself a couple of times to get the proper cadence.)

SEATED HAMSTRING/LOW-BACK STRETCH

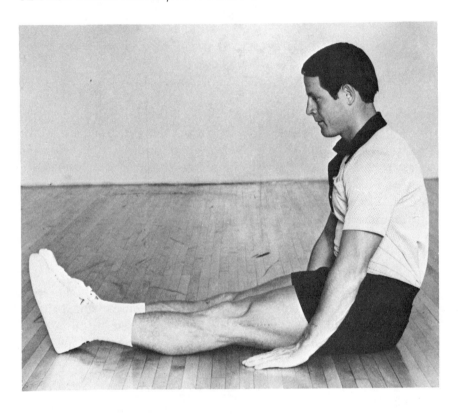

STARTING POSITION

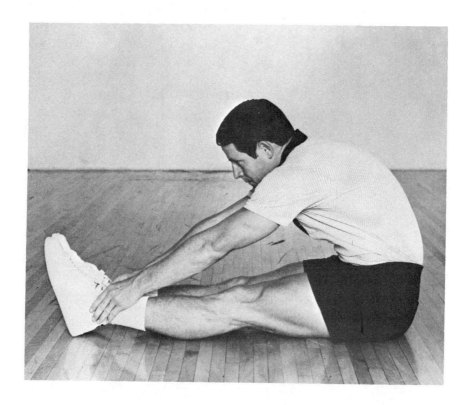

ACTION—
HOLD POSITION

2. *Seated Hamstring/Low-Back Stretch*

Purpose: To stretch the hamstrings and muscles of the lower back.

Starting Position: Sit on the floor with the legs straight and together.

Action: Bend forward, grasp the outer sides of the legs as close to the ankles as possible, and attempt to pull the shoulders downward. When you feel a stretch in the hamstrings, hold for the prescribed count. Keep the knees straight.

Cadence: Slow.

Progression: Start by holding for 15 seconds, and build up to 30 seconds. As flexibility improves, slide the hands closer to the ankles until you can grasp the outer edges of the feet. (*Note:* Concentrate on relaxing the quadriceps as the hamstrings are stretched.)

SEATED CROSSED-LEGS/HAMSTRING STRETCH

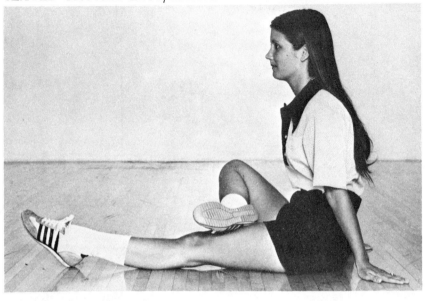

STARTING POSITION

ACTION—
HOLD POSITION

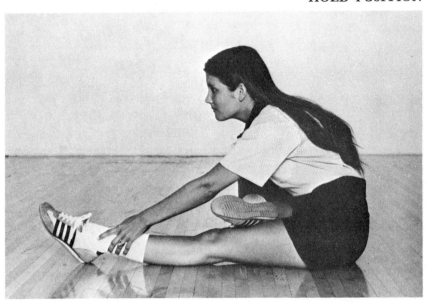

3. Seated Crossed-Legs/Hamstring Stretch

Purpose: To stretch the hamstrings on one leg at a time. Especially good for extremely tight hamstrings.

Starting Position: Sit on the floor with the left leg extended and the right leg bent so that the ankle is placed on top of the left thigh.

Action: Bend forward, grasp the extended leg with both hands, and hold at the point where you feel a stretch in the hamstrings. (*Note:* You may feel some of the stretch just below the back of the knee. That is because the hamstring muscles attach at that point.)

Cadence: Slow.

Progression: When you feel the stretch, hold for 15 seconds, and build up to 30 seconds. As your flexibility improves, grasp your leg nearer the ankle or grasp your toe. Repeat the exercise with the right leg extended. (*Note:* Concentrate on relaxing the quadriceps as the hamstrings are stretched.)

SQUAT-STRETCH FOR HAMSTRINGS

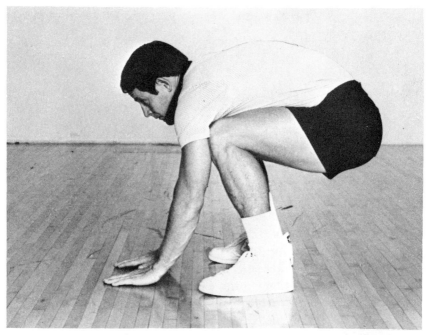

STARTING POSITION

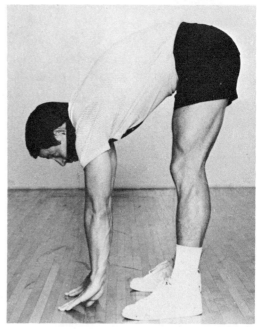

ACTION—
HOLD POSITION

4. Squat-Stretch for Hamstrings

Purpose: To stretch the hamstrings on both legs.

Starting Position: Squat with feet and knees together, and place hands on the floor in front of the feet.

Action: Keeping the hands on the floor, straighten the legs until a stretch is felt in the back of the legs. Hold for the prescribed count.

Cadence: Slow.

Progression: When you feel the stretch, hold for 15 seconds. Gradually increase the holding period for up to 30 seconds. (*Note:* Try to relax the quadriceps while stretching the hamstrings.)

QUADRICEPS/ILIOPSOAS STRETCH

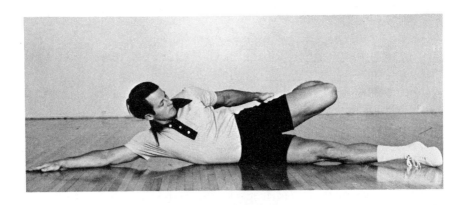

STARTING POSITION *AND*
ACTION-HOLD POSITION

5. Quadriceps/Iliopsoas Stretch

Purpose: To stretch the quadriceps and iliopsoas muscles.

Starting Position: Lie on the right side with the right leg extended and the left leg bent at the knee. Grasp the left foot between the ankle and the toes with the left hand.

Action: Pull the ankle backward while at the same time resisting the pull by pushing the instep into the palm of the hand until you feel a stretch in the quadriceps and in front of the hip. Hold for the prescribed count.

Cadence: Slow.

Progression: When the stretch is felt, hold for 15 seconds. Gradually increase the holding period for up to 30 seconds. Repeat using the right leg.

GROIN STRETCH

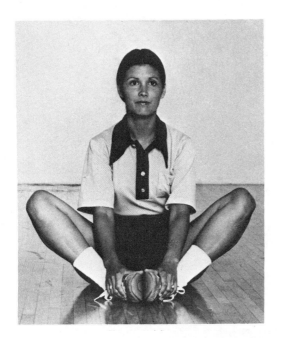

STARTING POSITION

ACTION—
HOLD POSITION

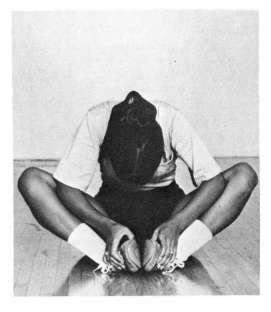

6. Groin Stretch

Purpose: To stretch the muscles in the groin area.

Starting Position: Sit on the floor with the soles of the feet together and the heels pulled close to the buttocks.

Action: Grasp your toes and pull the upper body forward until a stretch is felt in the groin area. Hold for the prescribed count.

Cadence: Slow.

Progression: When the stretch is felt, hold for 15 seconds. Gradually increase the holding period for up to 30 seconds.

FOOT AND ANKLE STRETCH

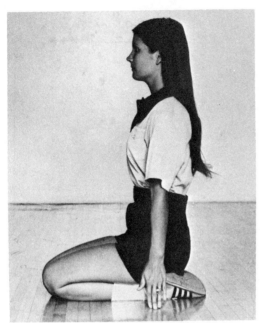

STARTING POSITION

ACTION—
HOLD POSITION

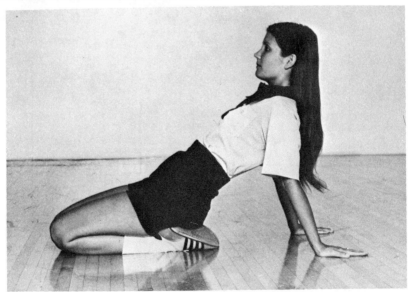

7. *Foot and Ankle Stretch*

Purpose: To stretch the muscles and tendons of the feet and ankles.

Starting Position: Kneel with knees and feet together and toes pointed to the rear.

Action: Slowly sit back, place hands on the floor behind you, and lower your shoulders until you feel a stretch in the feet and ankles. Hold for the prescribed count.

Cadence: Slow.

Progression: When you feel the stretch, hold for 15 seconds. Gradually increase the holding period for up to 30 seconds.

FEET OVER

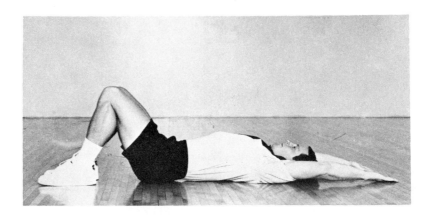

STARTING POSITION

ACTION—
HOLD POSITION

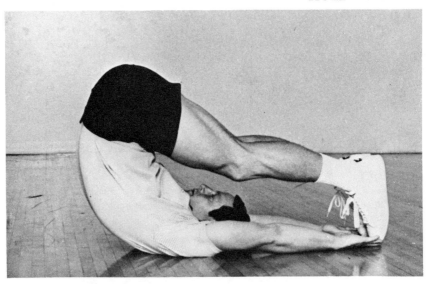

8. Feet Over

Purpose: To stretch the muscles of the upper and lower back and neck.

Starting Position: Lie on the floor with arms extended overhead and knees bent with feet on the floor.

Action: Slowly bring knees to the chest, continue rolling backward onto the shoulders, and extend the legs until the feet touch the floor above the head. Hold for the prescribed count.

Cadence: Slow.

Progression: When the toes touch the floor, hold for a count of 15. Gradually increase the holding period for up to 30 seconds.

SHOULDER/PECTORALS STRETCH

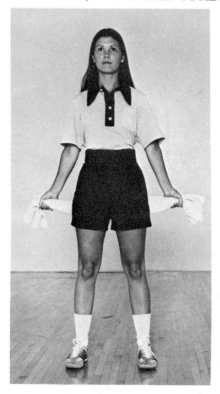

STARTING POSITION

ACTION—
HOLD POSITION

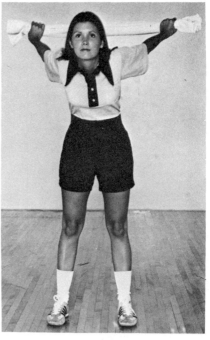

9. *Shoulder/Pectorals Stretch*

Purpose: To stretch the muscles of the shoulders and the pectoral
    muscles of the chest.
Starting Position: Stand holding a belt, rope, or towel behind the
    hips with the hands at shoulder width apart and elbows straight.
Action: Lift hands backward as high as possible until you feel the
    stretch in the shoulders and chest muscles. Thrust the hips
    forward to prevent bending forward.
Cadence: Slow.
Progression: When you feel the stretch, hold that position for a
    count of 15. Gradually increase the holding period for up to
    30 seconds.

SHOULDERS STRETCH

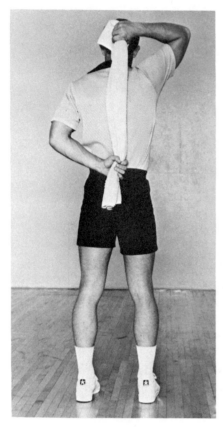

STARTING
POSITION

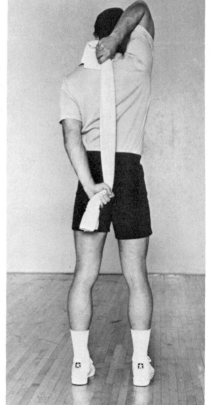

ACTION—COUNT 1
HOLD POSITION

10. *Shoulders Stretch*

Purpose: To stretch the muscles of the shoulders.

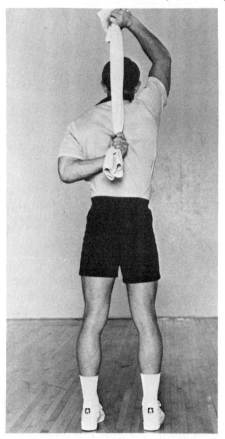

**ACTION–COUNT 2
HOLD POSITION**

Starting Position: Raise the right arm alongside the head, and bend
  the elbow so the right hand is behind the neck grasping one
  end of a towel. The left arm is bent up from behind the back,
  grasping the other end of the towel.
Action: Count 1: The left arm pulls down on the towel until a
  stretch is felt in the right shoulder. Hold for the specified
  count.
    Count 2: The right arm pulls up on the towel until the
  stretch is felt in the left shoulder. Hold for the specified count.
    Switch arms, and repeat with the left arm high and the right
  arm low.
Cadence: Slow.
Progressions: When you feel the stretch, hold for 15-second count
  at each position.

Chapter 11

The Winner's Circuit

West Point's largest gymnasium, about a city block in length and forty feet high, is in the Cadet Gymnasium Building. A balcony, with a 10-foot-wide running track, rings the gymnasium. During the day you will find men and women, ranging in age from late teens into their early sixties, in continual motion for a period of about twenty minutes. They stop at designated stations to perform specific exercises and then run to the next station. This is what we call circuit training.

The men and women are there voluntarily, except for those brought by coaches to maintain a team's General Athletic Fitness conditioning. Circuit training is an excellent conditioner, strongly and fully endorsed by the sports medicine establishment. It incorporates all the training and physical fitness components in a single workout, can be adapted to individual needs regardless of age and sex, and has enough built-in versatility to make the workout popular. It is the circuit concept that we've adapted for this book.

Circuit training surfaced in England about 1950, and within two years West Point had developed circuit programs. The basic idea is to lay out five to ten exercise stations on a circular path. A different exercise is performed at each station before a person runs on to the next. This combines both cardiorespiratory and skeletal muscle conditioning, two distinct categories, virtually unrelated.

The individual runs from station to station at a good, but not exhausting, pace and then performs the exercises as rapidly as possible for a specified number of minutes before moving on. As a result, circuit training is adjusted to the individual's current physical state. The stress is moderate but sufficient to maintain or improve fitness. Anyone can use it.

118

Circuits can be laid out in a gymnasium, along paths in the woods, on running tracks, in open fields, or around a city block. West Point has both indoor and outdoor circuits that have survived for nearly three decades because of their popularity. On the circuit during a typical noon period, you will find former college, professional, and world-class athletes and faculty members from the English, Mathematics, and Social Science departments. Later in the day, after classes, cadets on their own initiative run the circuit to keep in shape for their fitness tests and their favorite sports.

Circuit training appeals to faculty and students because it is comprehensive and time-efficient. The teacher gets finished in time for a quick lunch and his one o'clock class. The cadets, who are always stressed for time, can get on with their studies.

The Academy's indoor circuit has ten exercise stations on a track that takes 11.7 laps to the mile. After a warm-up during the first lap the individual stops at the first station to exercise for 1 minute and then runs slightly more than another lap at a comfortable speed before stopping and exercising again at the next station for 1 minute. A beginner in poor shape may take 22 to 25 minutes for a complete workout. By gradually reducing the lap time to 30 seconds per lap, anyone can get an excellent workout that covers all the physical components in 15 or 16 minutes.

The Winner's Circuit, so called because it develops a competitive edge, has been adapted for the weekender and has been so designed that it can be used almost anywhere, in the backyard, a vacant field, or, if you wish, your bedroom or living room. In the home, instead of actually running to develop cardiorespiratory conditioning, you may choose to run in place, jump rope, or ride a stationary bicycle.

The Winner's Circuit has been organized at three different levels. All have the same pattern:

Warm-up and flexibility exercises.

Circuit exercises.

Cool-down and flexibility exercises.

Although some flexibility exercises have been built into the circuit conditioning, especially in the lower levels, you begin with four warm-up/flexibility exercises to loosen muscles and tendons through stretching. Hold each of these exercises for the prescribed count as shown in the table on page 124. As you get the feel for this, try to relax other muscles while holding the stretch position. For instance, if stretching the hamstrings, concentrate on relaxing the quadriceps. This makes stretching more effective. If quadriceps are contracting, this prevents the full and complete stretching of the hamstrings. The same rule applies to other paired muscles of the body.

After completing the warm-up/stretching exercises, go immediately into the circuit. Begin with the prescribed time of cardiorespiratory exercise running, running in place, jumping rope, or riding a stationary bicycle. For example, at GAF Level I, Progression Step 1 (page 124), you start off with 30 seconds of cardiorespiratory (CR) conditioning and, without pausing, immediately go into the knee raising. After 15 repetitions, immediately go into another 30 seconds of CR conditioning before doing 15 repetitions of the trunk twister. Without pause, continue alternating the CR and muscle conditioning until you have completed all five muscle exercises, and then finish the circuit with a 1-minute bout of CR conditioning. Once the circuit is complete, go back to the flexibility/stretching exercises to cool off and bring your pulse down.

The above represents the minimum level of conditioning that is acceptable for the weekender who is participating only in light-activity sports. At the bottom of the table, you will find a category titled "Extra Edge." This is not necessarily required for your sport, but it will give you an additional competitive edge by improving your CR fitness.

If you go for the Extra Edge, there are several ways to work it into the schedule. It may precede or follow the circuit conditioning or be scheduled at a different time of the day. Or you may choose to do the circuit conditioning on three alternate days of the week, Monday, Wednesday, and Friday, and then work in the Extra Edge on Tuesday, Thursday, and Saturday with a complete rest on Sunday.

Listening to Body Talk

Your conditioning will improve faster if you exercise daily, but this is subject to the feedback you get from your muscles. If you are totally exhausted after completing the circuit, you should consider skipping it the following day. Sports research has taught us that when muscles are worked to total exhaustion, it takes about forty-eight hours to recover. On the other hand, this rule doesn't apply to CR conditioning. If possible, you should continue the running part of the program daily.

Tuning the Circuit to Your Intensity

Evaluate your intensity in competition. For example, it's generally agreed that we compete with less intensity as we get older. For that reason two competitors in their fifties will likely play tennis with less vigor than opponents who are younger. Consequently, an older person probably shouldn't condition to Level III. On the other hand, older persons who are unable to reach Step 3 of GAF Level I should limit themselves to a leisurely game of doubles. There are other factors that may limit intensity, such as being overfat, illness, or pregnancy. Still, none of these observations is intended by implication to compromise the basic theme of the book: If you want a competitive edge, you must condition yourself above the level of your play.

This Is Important

If you haven't been exercising regularly between weekend bouts of athletic activity, you should start with Progression Step 1, Level I, and stay with it for two weeks before going on to Step 2. Then spend two weeks in Step 2 before beginning Step 3. Continue to work up gradually to the level and step that are appropriate to your activity.

If you believe that you are in fair condition, you can begin at a higher level. Give it a try, but don't hesitate to drop back. In the long run you will make better progress through moderate stress.

If you are bedridden for several days or longer, pick up your circuit conditioning at a level lower than you have chosen for maintenance.

A Special Note to Women Edging Up

Fitness experts have learned that most men and women dislike the word "unisex" for reasons that would be better explored by a psychologist or sexologist. Therefore, the exercises are not called

unisex, but they are because we have made no special allowance
for women. The Academy has found that women can and should
undertake the same conditioning as men. Many women cadets do
fewer repetitions than the men or take more time, but you will find
women working the circuit alongside the men and receiving the
same valuable benefits.

Those Hell-born Push-ups

The demon who invented push-ups may never be identified, and
it's probably better that way. The push-up may be the most efficient
way to develop upper-torso strength in the home, but it is universally hated. If you can't do one push-up, let alone a dozen,
frustration reaches the boiling point. However, there's a reasonably
easy way to bring up your strength and ego to do full push-ups,
and this should have your earnest consideration because the push-up
is a very efficient way to develop the upper-torso strength that is
critical in sports activity.

A push-up must be done with straight legs and back. If you
can't do a single one off the floor, start by pushing off a wall from a
standing position. Gradually work your way down to a slightly
lower level, such as a highboy, bookcase, or upright piano. Then
move down to the level of a table or desk, about thirty inches off
the floor. You will then be lifting about 50 percent of your body
weight. When you have developed the strength to do repetitions
off a table, push off the end of a bed, which is about two feet off
the floor. You will be lifting about 60 percent of your weight.

Eventually you will be on the floor doing full push-ups. This
method follows the same principle of gradually increasing resistance
used by the Greek Milo when he began by carrying a newborn
heifer on his shoulder and continued until it was fully grown.
The same principle works with push-ups, and we know weekenders,
men and women, who have followed this procedure successfully.
When pushing off the floor, a woman lifts about 75 percent of her
weight; a man, about 76.5 percent. The difference is explained
by a woman's lower center of gravity.

One warning: The push-up that has become popular with
women, pushing off bent knees instead of the feet, is almost worth-
less because the woman is lifting less than 20 percent of body

weight. A woman using this exercise should move on to straight-leg push-ups.

Efficiency, Not Anxiety

In respect for the reader who is committed to his profession, we do not intend to abuse your time. All the exercises have been chosen for their efficiency. The program will take 20 to 30 minutes of your time, less as you get the swing of it. Furthermore, we suggest that when you can do the exercises automatically, about the time that the workout becomes boring, put your mind on something else. Just as it is possible to chew gum and think at the same time, you can exercise and think simultaneously—plan a speech, your work, a game plan or turn on the radio or TV.

You will progress more rapidly if you exercise daily, but if you miss a day, forget it. Ignore anxiety. Don't let it nag at you. However, you should exercise regularly on alternate days. And don't worry about that. After the first month, your body will virtually demand exercise—because it makes you feel better.

GAF LEVEL I

Light-Activity Sport—or If You Play a Moderate-Activity Sport Just for the Fun of It

	Progression Step 1	Progression Step 2	Progression Step 3
Warm-up/Flexibility			
	1. Achilles Stretch	Same exercises	Same exercises
	2. Seated Hamstring/Low-Back Stretch		
	9. Shoulder/Pectorals Stretch		
	7. Foot and Ankle Stretch		
	Hold for 15 seconds	Hold for 20 seconds	Hold for 30 seconds
	Then: 30 seconds cardiorespiratory conditioning	45 seconds cardiorespiratory conditioning	1:00 cardiorespiratory conditioning
Circuit Exercises			
	Abdomen—Knee Raiser—15 repetitions	20 repetitions	25 repetitions
	30 seconds cardiorespiratory conditioning	45 seconds cardiorespiratory conditioning	1:00 cardiorespiratory conditioning
	Trunk—Trunk Twister—15 repetitions	20 repetitions	25 repetitions
	30 seconds cardiorespiratory conditioning	45 seconds cardiorespiratory conditioning	1:00 cardiorespiratory conditioning

Thighs—Half Squat—15 repetitions	20 repetitions	25 repetitions
30 seconds cardiorespiratory conditioning	45 seconds cardiorespiratory conditioning	1:00 cardiorespiratory conditioning
Lower Legs—Toe Raiser—15 repetitions	20 repetitions	25 repetitions
30 seconds cardiorespiratory conditioning	45 seconds cardiorespiratory conditioning	1:00 cardiorespiratory conditioning
Arm/Shoulder—Modified Push-ups—15 repetitions (select your own start height)	20 repetitions	25 repetitions
1:00 cardiorespiratory conditioning	1:30 cardiorespiratory conditioning	2:00 cardiorespiratory conditioning

Cool-down/Flexibility

1, 2, 9, 7—Same as Warm-up/Flex above (Hold for 15 seconds)	Same exercises (Hold for 20 seconds)	Same exercises (Hold for 30 seconds)

Extra Edge

Run/walk 1 Mile 10 minutes	Run/walk 1 mile 9 minutes	Run/walk 1 mile 8 minutes

CIRCUIT EXERCISES
GAF LEVEL I

GAF LEVEL I

KNEE RAISER

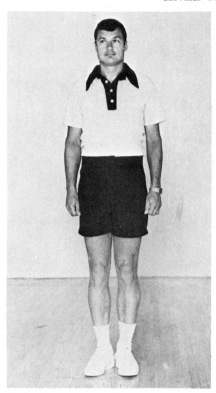

STARTING
POSITION

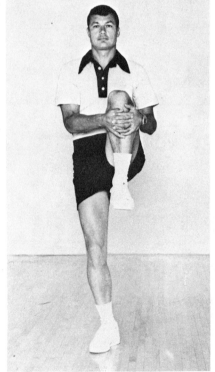

COUNT 1

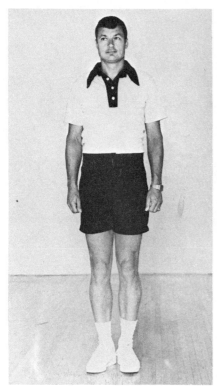

COUNT 2

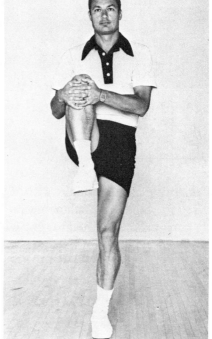

COUNT 3

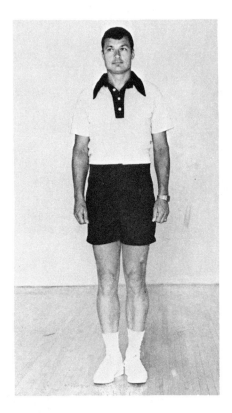

COUNT 4

Knee Raiser

Starting Position: Stand with feet together, arms at side, head up.
Action: Count 1: Balancing on the right leg, raise the left knee to
   its maximum height, grasp the leg at the shin with your hands,
   and pull it tightly into the body.
      Count 2: Return to the starting position.
      Count 3: Balancing on the left leg, raise the right knee to
   its maximum height, grasp the leg at the shin with your hands,
   and pull it tightly into the body.
      Count 4: Return to the starting position.
Cadence: Slow.

GAF LEVEL I

TRUNK TWISTER

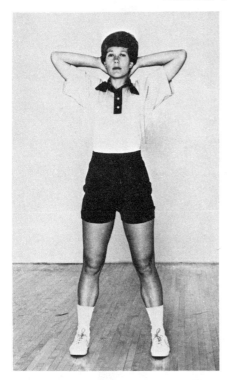

STARTING
POSITION

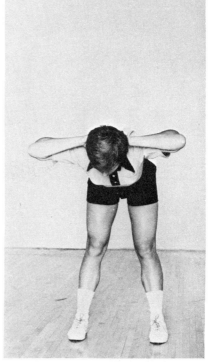

COUNT 1

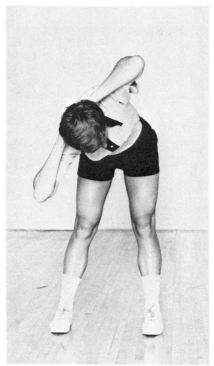

COUNT 2

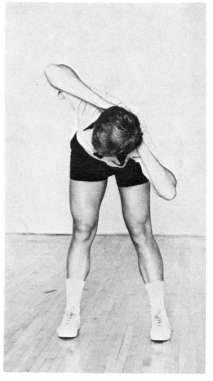

COUNT 3

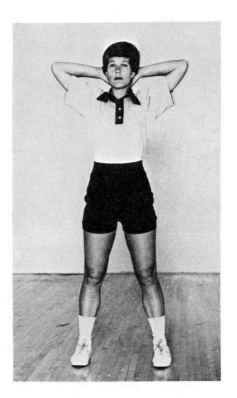

COUNT 4

Trunk Twister

Starting Position: Stand with feet separated about shoulder width, head up, hands interlaced behind the head, legs straight.
Action: Count 1: Bend forward to waist level.
   Count 2: Twist trunk to left, keeping elbows back.
   Count 3: Twist trunk to right, keeping elbows back.
   Count 4: Return to the starting position.
Cadence: Moderate to fast.

GAF LEVEL I

HALF SQUAT

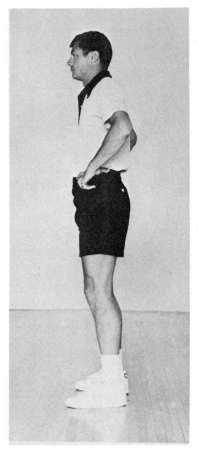

STARTING
POSITION

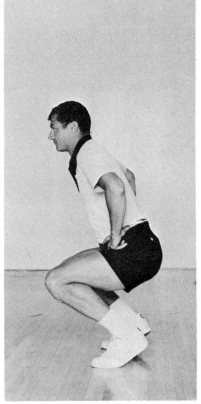

COUNT 1

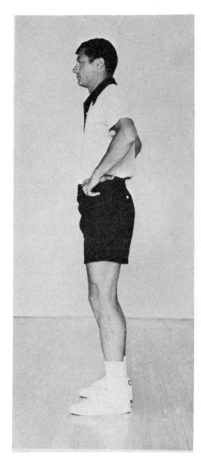

COUNT 2

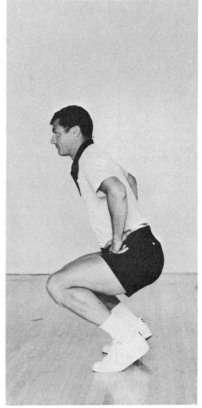

COUNT 3

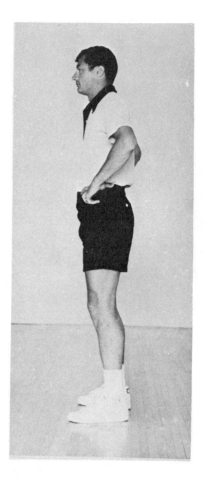

COUNT 4

Half Squat

Starting Position: Stand with feet spread about eight inches and
    hands on hips.
Action: Count 1: Bend knees to half-squat position until the
    thighs are parallel with the floor.
    Count 2: Return to the starting position.
    Count 3: Bend knees to half-squat position until the thighs
    are parallel with the floor.
    Count 4: Return to the starting position.
Cadence: Moderate to fast.

GAF LEVEL I

TOE RAISER

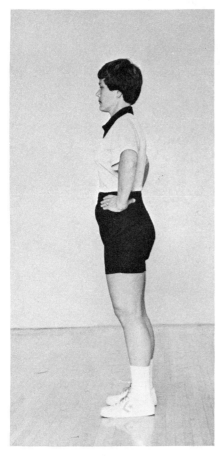

STARTING
POSITION

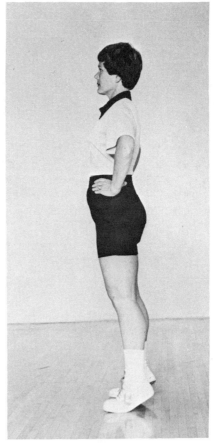

COUNT 1

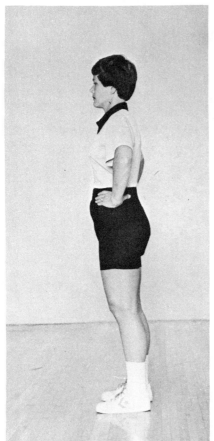

COUNT 2

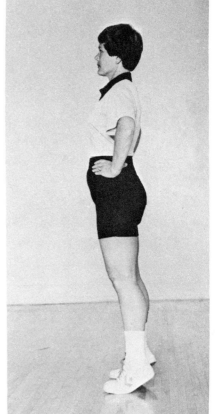

COUNT 3

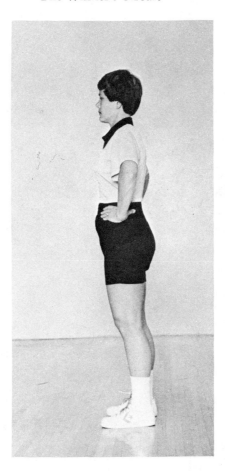

COUNT 4

Toe Raiser

Starting Position: Stand with feet together, hands on hips, head up.
Action: Count 1: Raise up on your toes as high as possible without losing balance.

Count 2: Return to the starting position.

Count 3: Raise up on your toes as high as possible without losing balance.

Count 4: Return to the starting position.
Cadence: Moderate.

GAF LEVEL I

MODIFIED PUSH-UPS

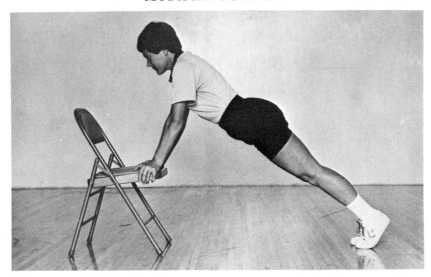

STARTING POSITION

COUNT 1

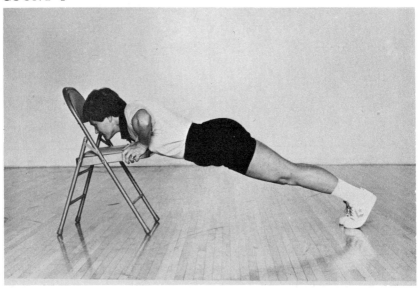

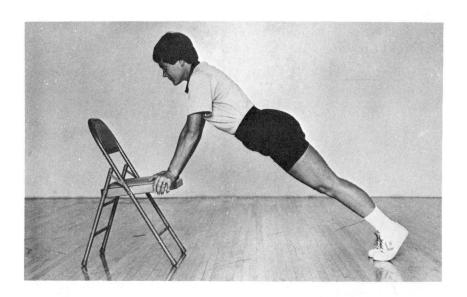

COUNT 2

COUNT 3

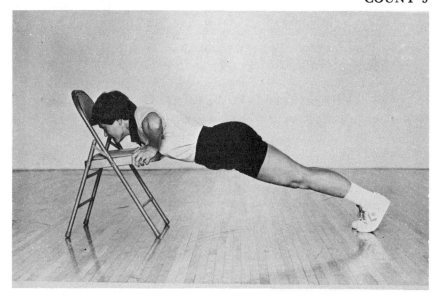

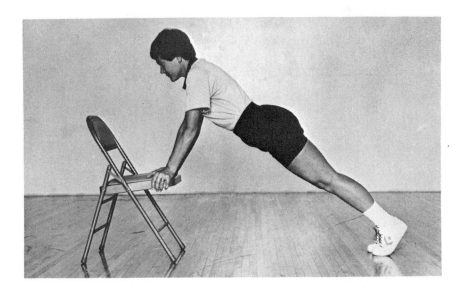

COUNT 4

Modified Push-ups

Starting Position: Place hands about shoulder width apart on the
    front edge of a heavy table or dresser (about three feet high)
    with the feet together and located approximately three-fourths
    of a body length away from the hands.
Action: Count 1: Keeping head up, bend your arms and lower
    your body until your chest touches the front edge of the
    dresser/table.
    Count 2. Push up, straightening your arms until you are
    back in the starting position.
    Count 3: Repeat Count 1.
    Count 4: Repeat Count 2.
Cadence: Moderate to fast.

GAF LEVEL II

Moderate-Activity Sport—or If You Play a Heavy-Activity Sport Just for the Fun of It

	Progression Step 1	Progression Step 2	Progression Step 3
Warm-up/Flexibility			
1. Achilles Stretch			
3. Seated Crossed-Legs/Hamstring Stretch	Same stretching exercises	Same stretching exercises	Same stretching exercises
10. Shoulders Stretch, with towel			
7. Foot and Ankle Stretch			
Hold for 15 seconds	Hold for 20 seconds	Hold for 30 seconds	
Then: 1:15 cardiorespiratory conditioning	1:30 cardiorespiratory conditioning	1:45 cardiorespiratory conditioning	
Circuit Exercises			
Abdomen—Bent Knee Curl—20 repetitions	25 repetitions	30 repetitions	
1:15 cardiorespiratory conditioning	1:30 cardiorespiratory conditioning	1:45 cardiorespiratory conditioning	
Trunk—Bend and Reach—20 repetitions	25 repetitions	30 repetitions	
1:15 cardiorespiratory conditioning	1:30 cardiorespiratory conditioning	1:45 cardiorespiratory conditioning	

Thighs/Hips/Buttocks—Squat Thrust—20 repetitions	25 repetitions	30 repetitions
1:15 cardiorespiratory conditioning	1:30 cardiorespiratory conditioning	1:45 cardiorespiratory conditioning
Lower Legs—Elevated Toe Raises—20 repetitions	25 repetitions	30 repetitions
1:15 cardiorespiratory conditioning	1:30 cardiorespiratory conditioning	1:45 cardiorespiratory conditioning
Arm/Shoulder—Push-ups—20 repetitions	25 repetitions	30 repetitions
2:30 cardiorespiratory conditioning	3:00 cardiorespiratory conditioning	4:00 cardiorespiratory conditioning

Cool-down/Flexibility

1, 3, 7, 10—Same as Warm-up/Flex above (Hold for 15 seconds)	Same exercises (Hold for 20 seconds)	Same exercises (Hold for 30 seconds)

Extra Edge

Run 1½ miles 14 minutes	Run 1½ miles 13 minutes	Run 1½ miles 12 minutes

CIRCUIT EXERCISES
GAF LEVEL II

GAF LEVEL II

BENT-KNEE CURL

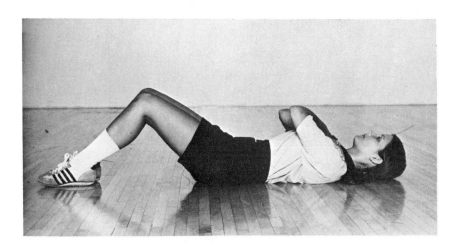

STARTING POSITION

COUNT 1

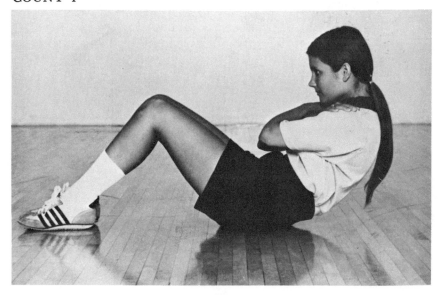

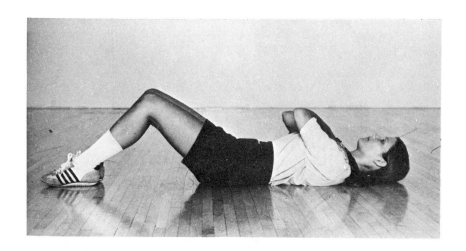

COUNT 2

COUNT 3

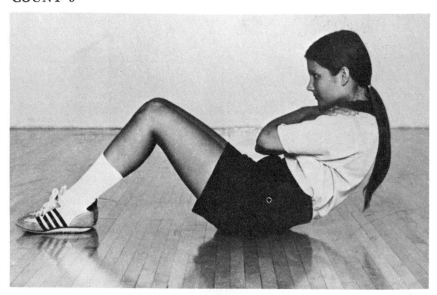

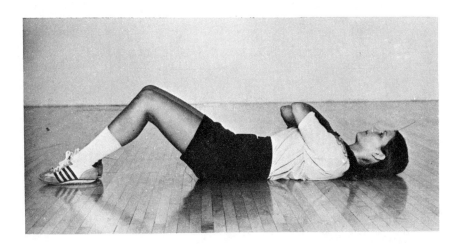

COUNT 4

Bent-Knee Curl

Starting Position: Lie on back with knees bent at an angle of 45
to 90 degrees, left hand on right shoulder and right hand on
left shoulder, with arms crossed over the chest.

Action: Count 1: Tucking chin into your chest, curl forward into
a half-sitting position until your shoulders are about one foot
off the floor. Hold for a count of 5 seconds.

Count 2: Slowly return to starting position.

Count 3: Repeat Count 1.

Count 4: Return to starting position.

Cadence: Slow.

GAF LEVEL II

BEND AND REACH

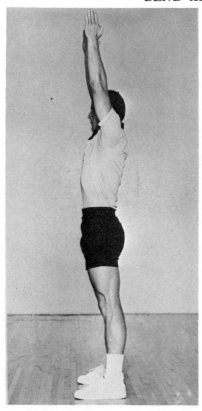

STARTING
POSITION

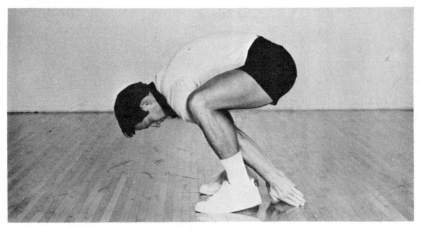

COUNT 1

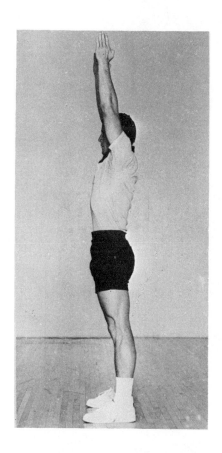

COUNT 2

COUNT 3

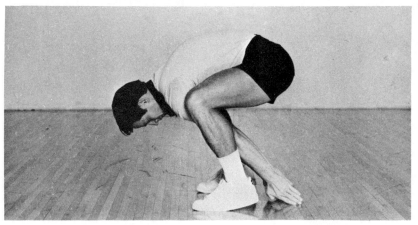

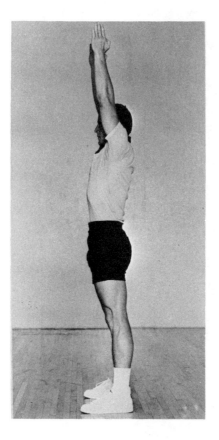

COUNT 4

Bend and Reach

Starting Position: Stand with feet separated shoulder width apart, arms straight and overhead.

Action: Count 1: Bend forward and extend arms between the legs, touching hands to the floor as far behind your heels as possible.

   Count 2: Return to starting position.

   Count 3: Repeat Count 1.

   Count 4. Return to starting position.

Cadence: Moderate to fast.

GAF LEVEL II

SQUAT THRUST

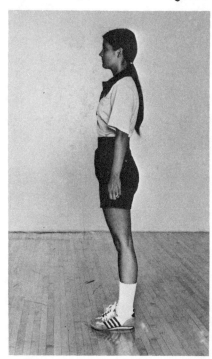

STARTING
POSITION

COUNT 1

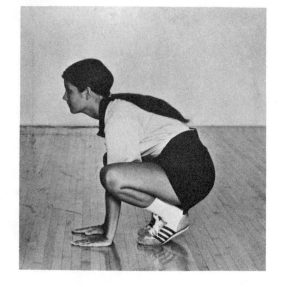

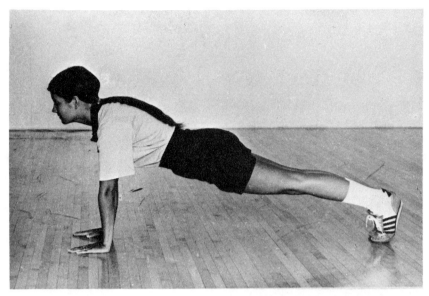

COUNT 2

COUNT 3

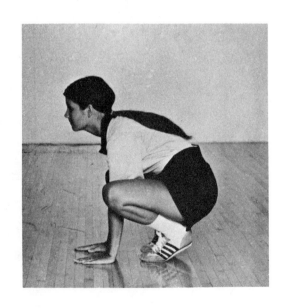

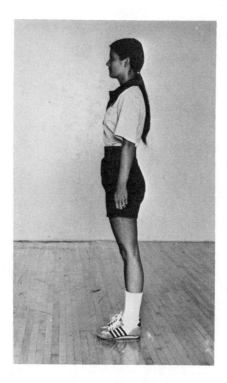

COUNT 4

Squat Thrust

Starting Position: Stand straight with feet together and arms at sides.

Action: Count 1: Squat and place hands on the floor with arms inside the knees.

　　Count 2: Extend legs to the rear to the front leaning rest position.

　　Count 3: Return to the full-squat position.

　　Count 4: Return to the standing position.

Cadence: Moderate to fast.

GAF LEVEL II

ELEVATED TOE RAISES

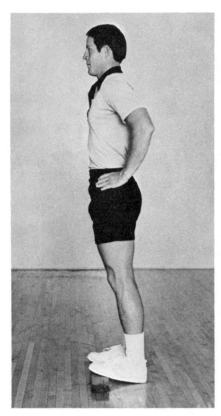

STARTING
POSITION

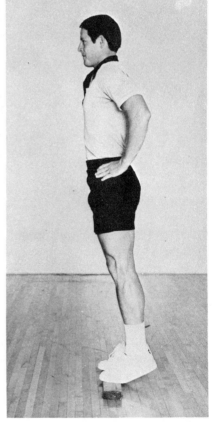

COUNT 1

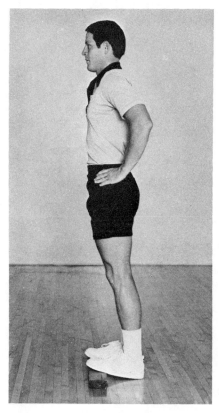

COUNT 2

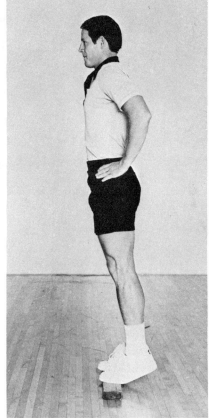

COUNT 3

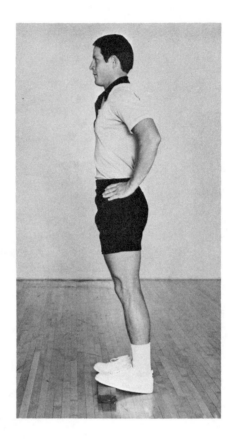

COUNT 4

Elevated Toe Raises

Starting Position: Stand with toes on a thick book or board with
heels on the floor and arms at your sides, hands on hips.

Action: Count 1: Raise up your toes as high as possible while
holding your balance.

Count 2: Return to starting position.

Count 3: Repeat Count 1.

Count 4: Return to starting position.

Cadence: Slow to moderate.

GAF LEVEL II

PUSH-UPS

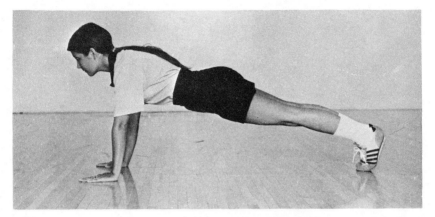

STARTING POSITION

COUNT 1

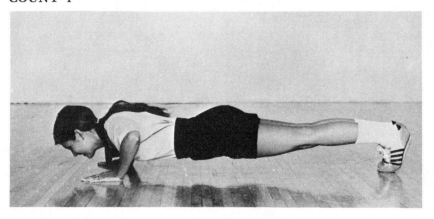

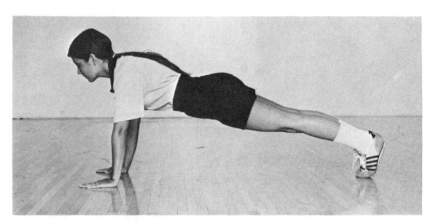

COUNT 2

COUNT 3

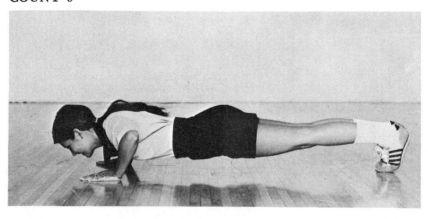

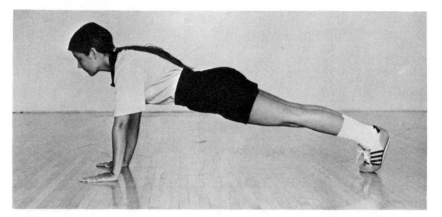

COUNT 4

Push-ups

Starting Position: Front leaning rest position with hands on floor, shoulder width apart, arms straight, body straight from shoulders to heels.

Action: Count 1: Bend arms and lower body while maintaining it in a straight line, until the chest touches the floor.

Count 2: Straighten arms, and return to the starting position.

Count 3: Repeat Count 1.

Count 4: Return to starting position.

Cadence: Moderate to fast.

GAF LEVEL III
(Heavy-Activity Sport)

Progression Step 1	Progression Step 2	Progression Step 3
Warm-up/Flexibility		
1. Achilles Stretch		
5. Quadriceps/Iliopsoas Stretch		
8. Feet Over		
9. Shoulder/Pectorals Stretch		
Hold for 15 seconds	Hold for 20 seconds	Hold for 30 seconds
	Same stretching exercises	Same stretching exercises
Then: 2:00 cardiorespiratory conditioning	2:30 cardiorespiratory conditioning	3:00 cardiorespiratory conditioning
Circuit Exercises		
Abdomen—Bent-Knee Sit-up—25 repetitions	30 repetitions	35 repetitions
2:00 cardiorespiratory conditioning	2:30 cardiorespiratory conditioning	3:00 cardiorespiratory conditioning
Trunk—Rowing—25 repetitions	30 repetitions	35 repetitions
2:00 cardiorespiratory conditioning	2:30 cardiorespiratory conditioning	3:00 cardiorespiratory conditioning

Thighs/Hips/Buttocks—Step-ups—25 repetitions	30 repetitions	35 repetitions
2:00 cardiorespiratory conditioning	2:30 cardiorespiratory conditioning	3:00 cardiorespiratory conditioning
Lower Legs—High Jumper—25 repetitions	30 repetitions	35 repetitions
2:00 cardiorespiratory conditioning	2:30 cardiorespiratory conditioning	3:00 cardiorespiratory conditioning
Arms/Shoulders—Eight Count Push-ups—10 repetitions	15 repetitions	20 repetitions
4:00 cardiorespiratory conditioning	5:00 cardiorespiratory conditioning	5:00 cardiorespiratory conditioning

Cool-down/Flexibility

1, 5, 8, 9—Same as Warm-up/Flex above (Hold for 15 seconds)	Same exercises (Hold for 20 seconds)	Same exercises (Hold for 30 seconds)

Extra Edge

Run 2 miles 18 minutes	Run 2 miles 17 minutes	Run 2 miles 16 minutes

CIRCUIT EXERCISES
GAF LEVEL III

GAF LEVEL III

BENT-KNEE SIT-UP

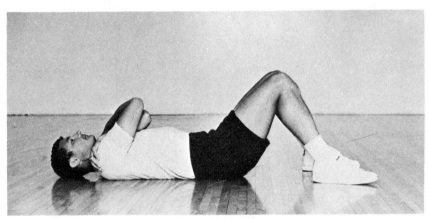

STARTING POSITION

COUNT 1

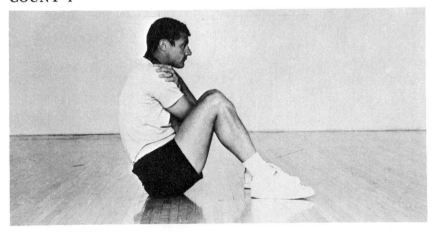

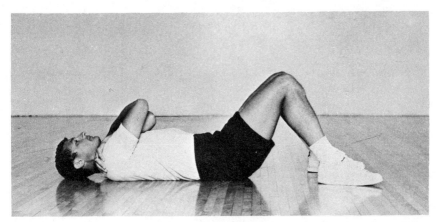

COUNT 2

COUNT 3

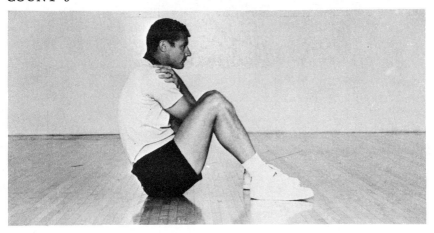

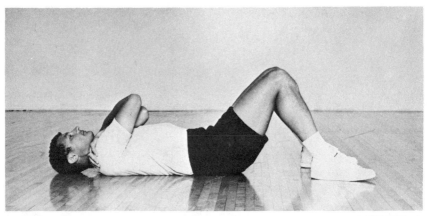

COUNT 4

Bent-Knee Sit-up

Starting Position: Lie on back with knees bent at an angle of 45 to 90 degrees, arms crossed with left hand on right shoulder and right hand on left shoulder.

Action: Count 1: Tuck chin to chest and curl forward as far as possible or until your arms touch your thighs.

    Count 2: Return to starting position.

    Count 3: Repeat Count 1.

    Count 4: Return to starting position.

Cadence: Moderate to fast.

GAF LEVEL III

ROWING

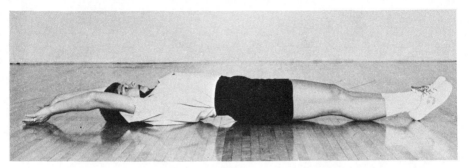

STARTING POSITION

COUNT 1

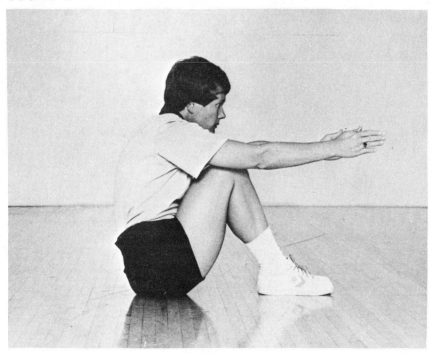

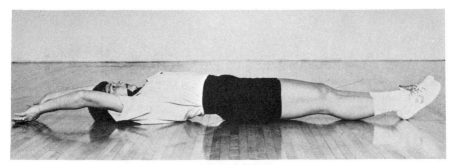

COUNT 2

COUNT 3

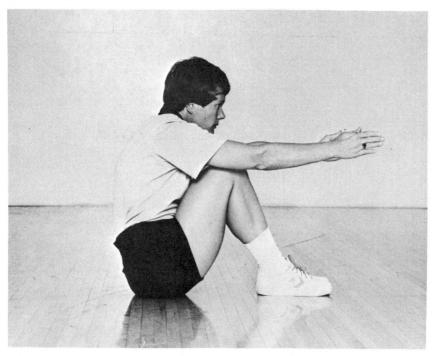

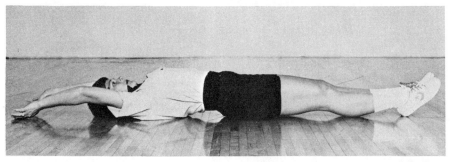

COUNT 4

Rowing

Starting Position: Lie on back with legs together and arms extended overhead.

Action: Count 1: Sit up and swing the arms over the head to a position parallel to the floor; at the same time bring your heels in close to your buttocks. Knees are together and inside the arms.

Count 2: Return to starting position.

Count 3: Repeat Count 1.

Count 4: Return to starting position.

Cadence: Moderate to fast.

GAF LEVEL III

STEP-UPS

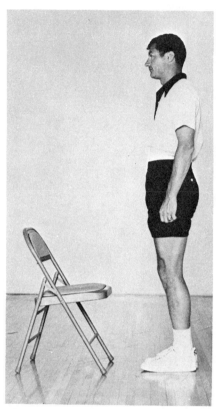

STARTING
POSITION

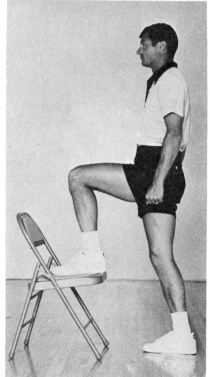

COUNT 1

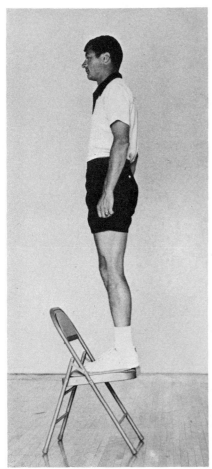

COUNT 2

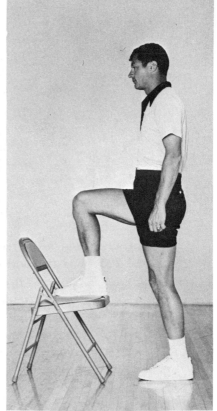

COUNT 3

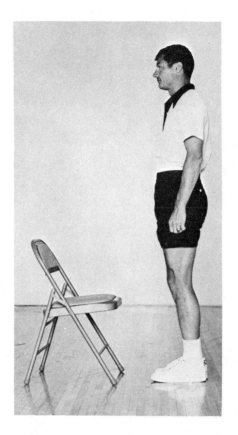

COUNT 4

Step-ups

Starting Position: Stand with feet together in front of a sturdy
    chair or a box or at the bottom of the stairs.
Action: Count 1: Step up with the left foot on the chair.
        Count 2: Bring your right foot up beside the left foot.
        Count 3: Lower your left foot back to the floor.
        Count 4: Lower your right foot back to the floor, returning
    to the starting position.
Cadence: Moderate to fast.

GAF LEVEL III

HIGH JUMPER

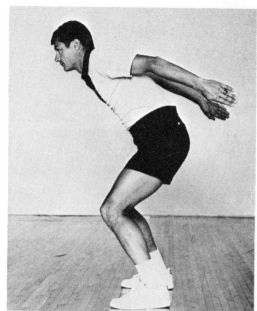

**STARTING
POSITION**

COUNT 1

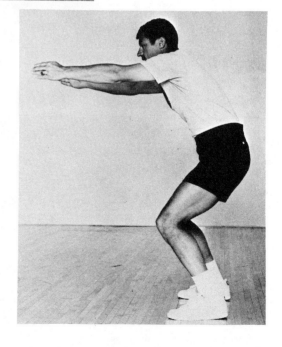

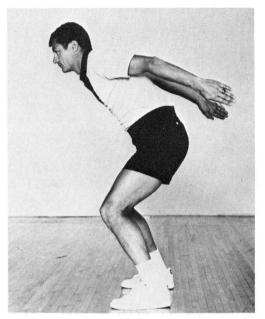

COUNT 2

COUNT 3

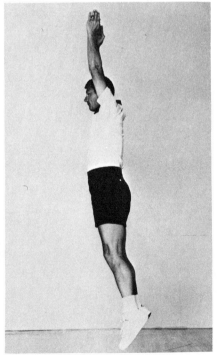

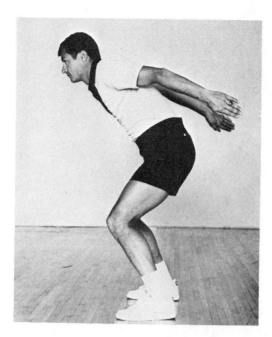

COUNT 4

High Jumper

Starting Position: Spread feet shoulder width apart with knees slightly flexed and the arms extended to the rear with palms facing.

Action: Count 1: Take a slight crow hop, while at the same time swinging the arms forward to a position parallel to the ground at shoulder height.

Count 2: Take another crow hop, and return to the starting position.

Count 3: Swing the arms vigorously overhead, and jump as high as possible. Look at your hands as you jump.

Count 4: Take another crow hop, and return to the starting position.

Cadence: Moderate to fast.

GAF LEVEL III

EIGHT-COUNT PUSH-UP

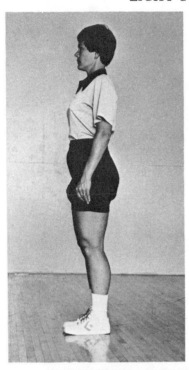

STARTING
POSITION

COUNT 1

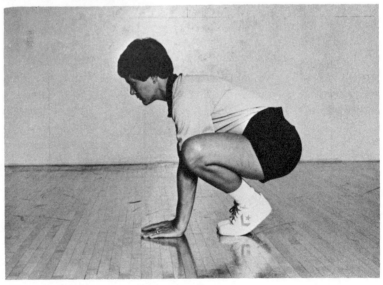

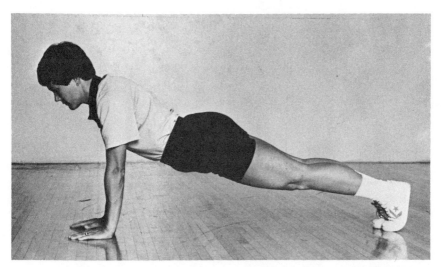

COUNT 2

COUNT 3

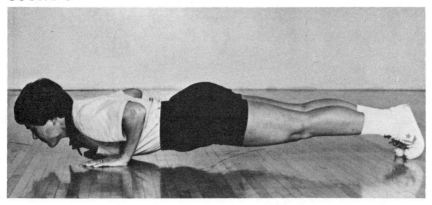

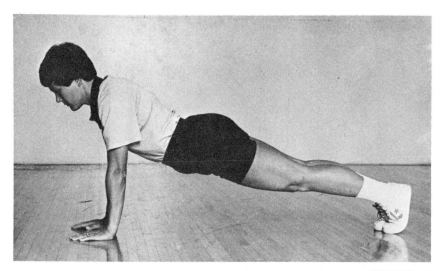

COUNT 4

COUNT 5

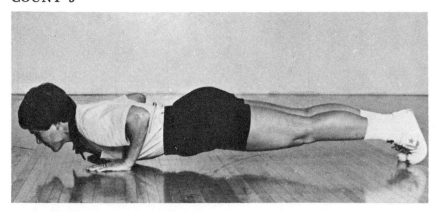

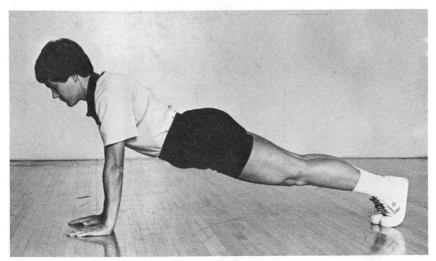

COUNT 6

COUNT 7

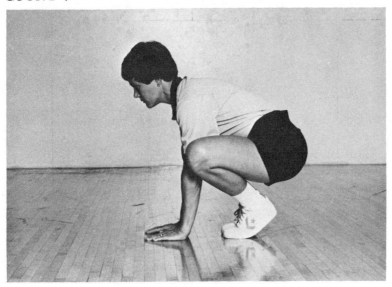

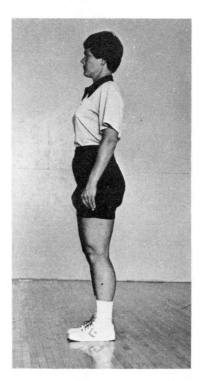

COUNT 8

Eight-Count Push-up

Starting Position: Stand with feet together, arms at sides, head up.
Action: Count 1: Squat down. Place palms flat on the floor about
    shoulder width apart, arms inside knees.
        Count 2: Thrust legs backward into front leaning position.
        Count 3: Bend arms, lowering body until chest touches
    floor.
        Count 4: Push up to front leaning rest position.
        Count 5: Repeat Count 3.
        Count 6: Repeat Count 4.
        Count 7: Return to squatting position.
        Count 8: Return to starting position.
Cadence: Moderate to fast.

PART III

Body Parts

Their Care and Maintenance

Chapter 12

Keeping It All Together

All of us—professional and amateur—are born with standard body parts. How we use or abuse these parts accounts for our performance. Health experts suggest that Americans take better care of their automobiles and pets than of their own bodies. Although this may be true of the sedentary population, weekend athletes are more likely to suffer biomechanical problems for a lack of information.

Weekenders don't know how to prevent injury and biomechanical inefficiency. Worse, when an injury occurs, there are few physicians who understand the physical and psychological nature of an athlete's frustration. Told to hibernate by a physician, the weekend athlete experiences a characteristic malaise. With inactivity, a certain psychological tone is lost. Weekenders call this the stir-crazies. Some say to hell with it, play hurt, and worsen the injury.

One weekend athlete, a physician, told us, "In the past, when someone came to me with a sport-related injury, I'd tell the patient to abstain from physical activity. Maybe I'd tape up the injured part and recommend soakings, but the prescription was 'rest, rest, rest,' and I guess that they used to hate me. I didn't understand what it was all about until I became a squash addict about three years ago. Now I can appreciate what it's like to be sidelined and how important it is to be active."

Keeping the hurt person active is basic policy at West Point. At the Academy a staff of trained sports medicine physicians gives the injured cadet a list of "what you can do" and "what you can't do." The exercise physiologists prescribe conditioning to maintain strength and flexibility in the well part of the body and exercises to bring the injured part back to normal. This is one of the major advances in sports medicine that sports research has to offer the general public.

Injuries and the SAPs—stiffness, aches, and pains—and losing are seldom related to basic health. The usual cause is biomechanical inefficiency, including muscular imbalance, poor form, a lack of flexibility, a racquet or ball held incorrectly or foot pronation. An analogy would be an automobile with a finely tuned (healthy) engine but with wheels out of alignment or brakes worn unevenly or any other defective part that causes erratic performance.

What follows is information about your body that relates to the efficient use of its parts—and how to maintain and, when necessary, recondition those parts.

The Active Body—An Overview

Sports are a natural function of the body. The activity puts the body to work. The game then becomes a challenge of strength, balance, endurance, motion, acumen, agility, dexterity, coordination, and joy.

The body is an interesting phenomenon, a wonder, in fact. The foundation is the skeletal-muscular system with 206 bones and more than 650 different muscles. The adjoining illustration of a skeleton shows the front and back view of a man's bones. Although the size of a woman's bones differs, the specific functions of the skeletal-muscular systems are the same. The skeleton itself provides:

1. The form and shape of the body.

2. A frame to help support the body's weight and mass against the pull of gravity. The frame is jointed to allow the body to move. It is given support by properly toned muscles and ligaments.

3. Protection and support for such vital and often delicate organs as the brain, trachea, spinal cord, lungs, heart, stomach, kidney, liver.

4. A storehouse within the bones for minerals and a factory that manufactures red blood cells and some kinds of white blood cells.

5. Bone surface for the attachment of the ligaments and tendons of the muscle groups.

Although bones maintain the rigidity, muscles supply the sup-

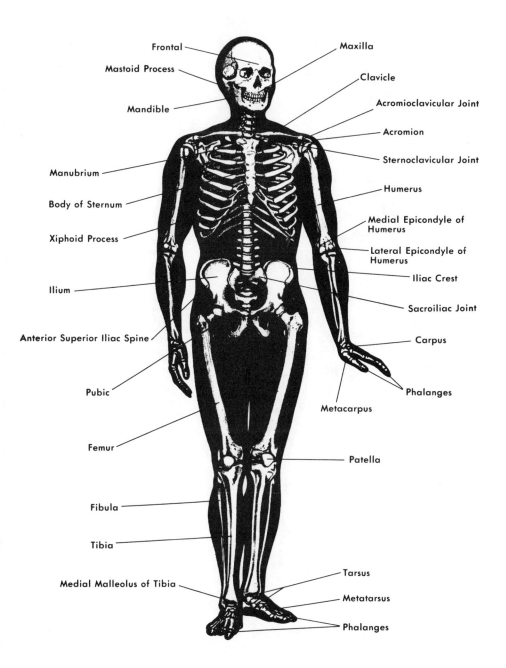

Frontal

Mastoid Process

Mandible

Manubrium

Body of Sternum

Xiphoid Process

Ilium

Anterior Superior Iliac Spine

Pubic

Femur

Fibula

Tibia

Medial Malleolus of Tibia

Maxilla

Clavicle

Acromioclavicular Joint

Acromion

Sternoclavicular Joint

Humerus

Medial Epicondyle of Humerus

Lateral Epicondyle of Humerus

Iliac Crest

Sacroiliac Joint

Carpus

Phalanges

Metacarpus

Patella

Tarsus

Metatarsus

Phalanges

1. FRONT SKELETAL VIEW

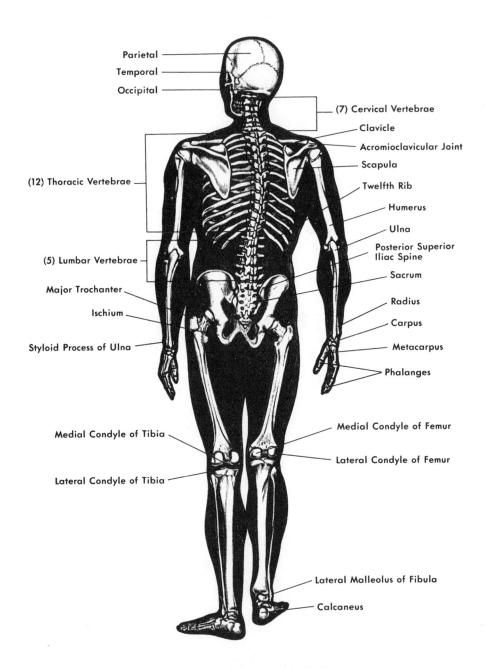

Parietal
Temporal
Occipital
(7) Cervical Vertebrae
Clavicle
Acromioclavicular Joint
Scapula
Twelfth Rib
Humerus
Ulna
Posterior Superior Iliac Spine
Sacrum
(12) Thoracic Vertebrae
Radius
Carpus
(5) Lumbar Vertebrae
Metacarpus
Major Trochanter
Phalanges
Ischium
Styloid Process of Ulna
Medial Condyle of Tibia
Medial Condyle of Femur
Lateral Condyle of Femur
Lateral Condyle of Tibia
Lateral Malleolus of Fibula
Calcaneus

2. BACK SKELETAL VIEW

port, just as hundreds of guy ropes support the tent poles and canvas in the big top.

Figures 3 and 4 (pages 184-185) show the front and rear views of some of the muscle groups and identify the actions that each group performs. Muscles work only when contracting. When the flexors contract, the joint bends; when the extensors contract, the joint straightens. When one group contracts, the other relaxes. This is the biomechanic binary system that performs all the complex, diverse, intricate fluid movements of which the jointed body is capable.

Sports research has identified the flow of motion through the different parts of the body as the athlete begins, follows through, and completes a specific sports action, such as throwing, kicking, jumping, vaulting, hitting, and running.

Generally in sports research the body movement is studied in halves: the upper body and the lower body. Aesthetically the better half may be in the eyes of the viewer, but from the viewpoint of the biomechanist it's the lower half that requires more tender loving care.

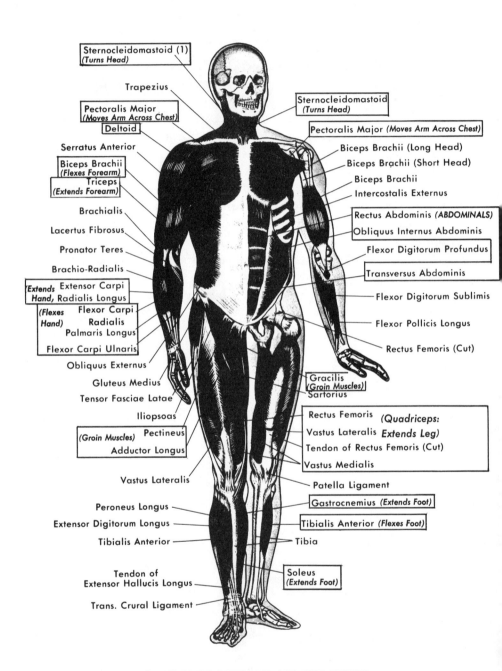

Sternocleidomastoid (1)
(Turns Head)

Trapezius

Pectoralis Major
(Moves Arm Across Chest)

Deltoid

Serratus Anterior

Biceps Brachii
(Flexes Forearm)

Triceps
(Extends Forearm)

Brachialis

Lacertus Fibrosus

Pronator Teres

Brachio-Radialis

(Extends Extensor Carpi
Hand) Radialis Longus

(Flexes Flexor Carpi
Hand) Radialis

Palmaris Longus

Flexor Carpi Ulnaris

Obliquus Externus

Gluteus Medius

Tensor Fasciae Latae

Iliopsoas

(Groin Muscles) Pectineus

Adductor Longus

Vastus Lateralis

Peroneus Longus

Extensor Digitorum Longus

Tibialis Anterior

Tendon of
Extensor Hallucis Longus

Trans. Crural Ligament

Sternocleidomastoid
(Turns Head)

Pectoralis Major (Moves Arm Across Chest)

Biceps Brachii (Long Head)

Biceps Brachii (Short Head)

Biceps Brachii

Intercostalis Externus

Rectus Abdominis (ABDOMINALS)

Obliquus Internus Abdominis

Flexor Digitorum Profundus

Transversus Abdominis

Flexor Digitorum Sublimis

Flexor Pollicis Longus

Rectus Femoris (Cut)

Gracilis
(Groin Muscles)
Sartorius

Rectus Femoris

Vastus Lateralis

Tendon of Rectus Femoris (Cut)

Vastus Medialis

Patella Ligament

Gastrocnemius (Extends Foot)

Tibialis Anterior (Flexes Foot)

Tibia

Soleus
(Extends Foot)

(Quadriceps:
Extends Leg)

3. FRONT MUSCULATURE VIEW

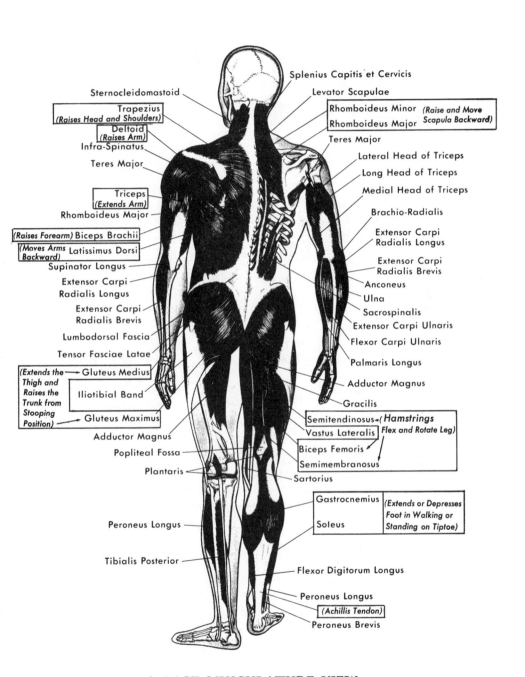

Splenius Capitis et Cervicis

Sternocleidomastoid

Levator Scapulae

Trapezius
(Raises Head and Shoulders)

Rhomboideus Minor (Raise and Move
Rhomboideus Major Scapula Backward)

Deltoid
(Raises Arm)

Infra-Spinatus

Teres Major

Teres Major

Lateral Head of Triceps

Long Head of Triceps

Medial Head of Triceps

Triceps
(Extends Arm)

Brachio-Radialis

Rhomboideus Major

Extensor Carpi
Radialis Longus

(Raises Forearm) Biceps Brachii

Extensor Carpi
Radialis Brevis

(Moves Arms Latissimus Dorsi
Backward)

Anconeus

Supinator Longus

Ulna

Extensor Carpi
Radialis Longus

Sacrospinalis

Extensor Carpi Ulnaris

Extensor Carpi
Radialis Brevis

Flexor Carpi Ulnaris

Lumbodorsal Fascia

Palmaris Longus

Tensor Fasciae Latae

Adductor Magnus

(Extends the → Gluteus Medius
Thigh and
Raises the
Trunk from
Stooping
Position)

Gracilis

Iliotibial Band

Semitendinosus (Hamstrings
Flex and Rotate Leg)

Vastus Lateralis

Gluteus Maximus

Biceps Femoris

Adductor Magnus

Semimembranosus

Popliteal Fossa

Sartorius

Plantaris

Gastrocnemius (Extends or Depresses
Foot in Walking or
Standing on Tiptoe)

Soleus

Peroneus Longus

Tibialis Posterior

Flexor Digitorum Longus

Peroneus Longus

(Achillis Tendon)

Peroneus Brevis

4. BACK MUSCULATURE VIEW

Chapter 13

The Lower Body and Its Best Parts

Sports research finds that the lower extremities of the body are most likely to be injured in either athletic participation or routine, everyday life. The explanation is biological evolution, which brought us to an upright posture and bipedal locomotion and thus placed an unusual burden on the feet, ankles, lower legs, knees, and thighs.

The lower body has two primary responsibilities, weight bearing and propulsion, and at the bottom of it are the feet, the mechanism for weight distribution when we are standing or moving—walking, running, jumping, dodging, pivoting, and the multiple of other movements that occur during normal sports activities.

The Foot, Bless It

When George Sheehan, runner, physician, and philosopher, visited West Point, he noted, "When an athlete, especially a runner, complains about pains anywhere from the lower back down, you should look first to the feet as the source of the trouble."

Dr. Sheehan's experience is virtually true of the clinical experience of podiatrists throughout the country. Whether the patient's pain is in the hips, knees, ankles, or lower back, the primary cause may be in the functioning of the foot.

If you look at Figures 5 and 6 (page 187), you will see that the foot has twenty-six bones which make up interconnecting arches. Not only do ligaments connect the bones, but some have the additional task of maintaining the arches. The longitudinal arch which extends lengthwise is, in fact, a double arch, one long and one short. The transverse metatarsal arch extends across the ball of the foot from one metatarsal bone to the other.

186

THE BONES OF THE FEET

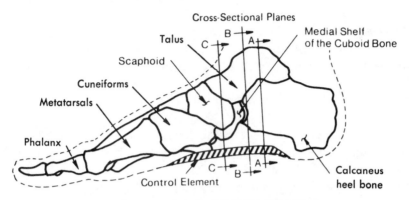

Cross-Sectional Planes

Talus

Scaphoid

Cuneiforms

Metatarsals

Phalanx

Medial Shelf
of the Cuboid Bone

Calcaneus
heel bone

Control Element

5. MEDIAL SIDE—RIGHT FOOT

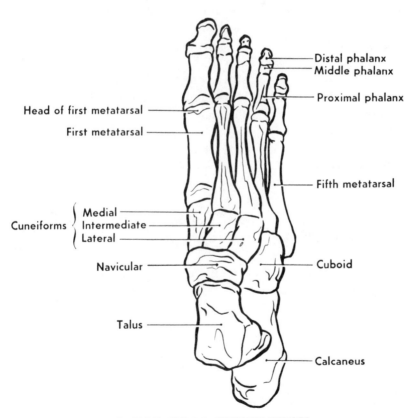

Distal phalanx
Middle phalanx

Proximal phalanx

Head of first metatarsal

First metatarsal

Fifth metatarsal

Cuneiforms { Medial
Intermediate
Lateral

Navicular

Cuboid

Talus

Calcaneus

6. TOP VIEW—RIGHT FOOT

Proper functioning and adequate development of the muscles, tendons, and ligaments of the foot are important for everyone but especially for the athlete. Not surprisingly when a sedentary person decides to get into shape for any physical activity, the first part of the body to complain is the feet. People talk about other aspects of their body when they should have their feet in their mouths.

Movements of the Foot

It's very important to keep the foot's muscles strong and its tendons and ligaments supple because the foot has a lot more going than you realize by merely watching a shoe rise and fall. In fact, the foot has eight different movements that are normal, and it might be worthwhile to take off a shoe and try these:

1. Dorsal Flexion: Movement of the top of the foot upward and toward the shin.
2. Plantar Flexion: Movement of the sole of the foot downward.
3. Abduction: Movement of the toes outward.
4. Adduction: Movement of the toes inward.
5. Eversion: Turning the sole of the foot outward with the weight bearing on the inner edge of the foot.
6. Inversion: Turning the sole inward with the weight bearing on the outer edge of the foot.
7. Toe Flexion: Curl toes down toward the floor.
8. Toe Extension Curl toes upward.

Practicing the above movements exercises the muscles, tendons, and ligaments and will help prepare the feet for strenuous activity.

MOVEMENTS OF THE FOOT

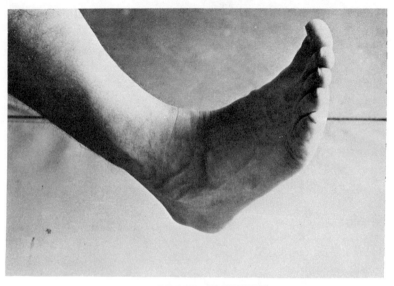

1. DORSAL FLEXION

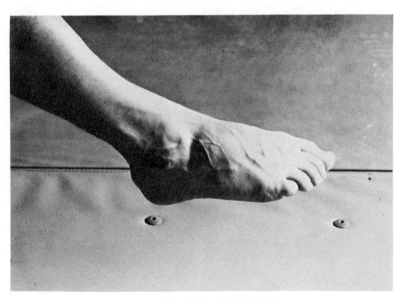

2. PLANTAR FLEXION

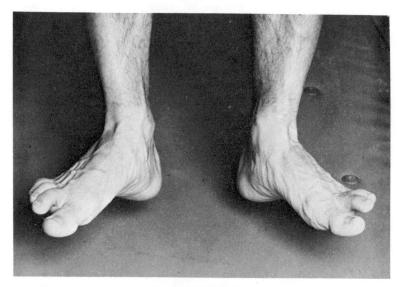

3. ABDUCTION

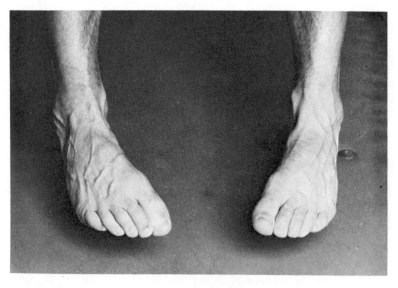

4. ADDUCTION

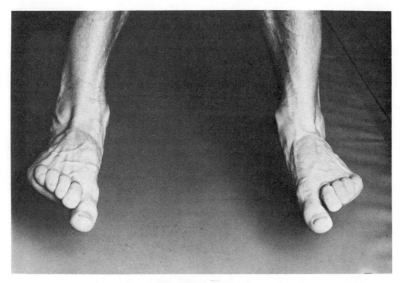

5. EVERSION

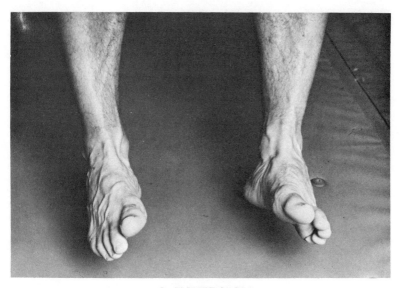

6. INVERSION

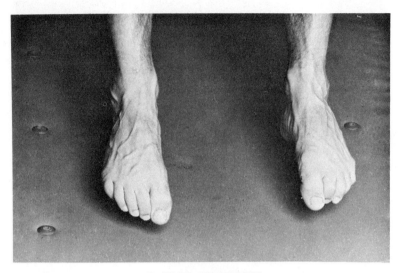

7. TOE FLEXION

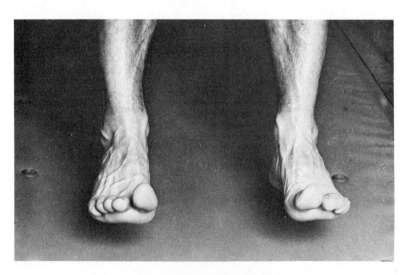

8. TOE EXTENSION

Common Causes of Foot Injury/Pain

Obviously, if we remember that the feet work on muscles just like a pitching or serving arm, we know the value of getting feet in shape with muscle conditioning when going from a sedentary life into sports activity. It's something for the active weekend athlete to keep in mind when returning to a seasonal sport. The exercises for the feet are a part of the General Athletic Fitness conditioning. The GAF at all three levels plus the foot movements already explained will help the weekender to condition the feet progressively.

Other factors that cause weak, sore, or injured feet include congenital defects, what we once called flat feet or high arches. These problems can be corrected by using properly fitted arch supports or orthodics prepared by a podiatrist.

The other major factor in foot fatigue and injury, a very common problem, is the improper placement of feet when you walk, run, and play. A biomechanist would tell you that your wheels need to be realigned.

Years ago we talked about kids who ran with their toes turned in as being pigeon-toed and those with toes turned out as being duck-footed. Now we describe the waddling walker as being splay-footed, and there are more splay-footed than pigeon-toed people in the world. Invariably, when a new class of cadets arrives at West Point, the few who have difficulty running and keeping up with their classmates run splay-footed. This seems especially true of large people, noticeably football linemen.

Toe in and toe out, pigeon or duck, we are talking not about congenital defects but about bad habits that lead to improper foot placement, that can be corrected, and it's worth the effort. Both bad habits decrease efficiency in movement. Toe out causes the weight stress to ride through the inside of the foot during propulsion instead of through the great toe. Similarly, excessive toe in means the weight stress, or line of propulsion, rides through the shorter and smaller outside toes. The correct stress line as the foot moves forward would run from the outside third of the heel at a slight angle along the bottom of the foot to a point just to the inside of the great toe.

The toe-in, toe-out positions not only are inefficient but also may be the cause of such injuries as stress fractures of the metatarsals, Achilles tendinitis, or pains in the calves, shin, and knees.

FOOT PLACEMENT AND STRESS LINES

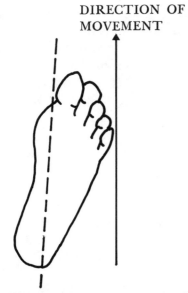

DIRECTION OF
MOVEMENT

STRESS LINE FOR *TOE-OUT*
OR DUCK-FOOTED
WALK/RUN

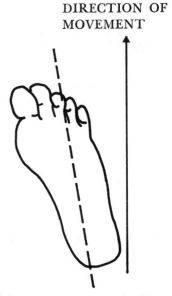

DIRECTION OF
MOVEMENT

STRESS LINE FOR *TOE-IN*
OR PIGEON-TOED
WALK/RUN

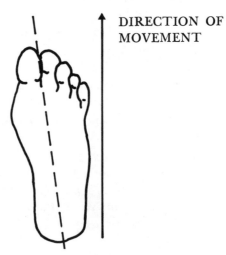

DIRECTION OF
MOVEMENT

STRESS LINE FOR *PROPER*
FOOT PLACEMENT

Prevention/Correction of Improper Foot Placement

The best time to correct foot placement is at a young age, and parents should look to this instead of assuming that everyone automatically learns to walk or run properly. Read on to see how to help your children. For the weekend adult athlete there are simple methods that can help correct foot placement without causing any pain. It merely takes concentration and patience.

Begin by observing that in the illustration on page196, the outside edges of the feet are parallel. As you look down at your own feet in this position, your toes will appear to be slightly turned in. But that is because of the shape of your feet.

When standing, walking, or running, practice placing your feet in the manner illustrated. It is the most effective method of propulsion. As part of the preseason practice, coaches should have athletes, especially the young ones, practice form running by running in slow motion. During this practice, concentrate on proper foot placement as an important factor in correcting running form. Weekend athletes should do the same.

To convince yourself of the importance of proper foot placement, try this:

Stand with your toes turned out and do a half squat. Note that your knees, when bending, end up in the same direction that your toes are pointing.

Now try the same half squat with your toes pointed in. Again your knees follow the direction of the toes.

Finally, try the half squat with the outside edges of your feet parallel. Your knees will point straight ahead, as they should be doing when you are walking or running. When knees are pointed incorrectly, out or in, undue stress is being placed on the joint, and this is a source of pain and strain.*

---

* One weekender believes that he helped correct his toe out by riding a stationary bicycle daily. If you try this, ride with the balls of your feet on the pedals, give your legs a full stretch, and every few minutes shout, "Hi-ho, Silver."

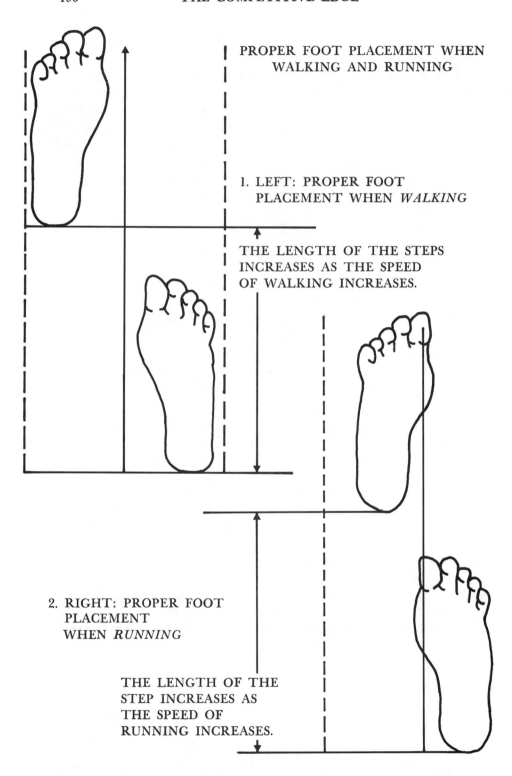

PROPER FOOT PLACEMENT WHEN
WALKING AND RUNNING

1. LEFT: PROPER FOOT
   PLACEMENT WHEN *WALKING*

THE LENGTH OF THE STEPS
INCREASES AS THE SPEED
OF WALKING INCREASES.

2. RIGHT: PROPER FOOT
   PLACEMENT
   WHEN *RUNNING*

THE LENGTH OF THE
STEP INCREASES AS
THE SPEED OF
RUNNING INCREASES.

WHY PROPER FOOT PLACEMENT?

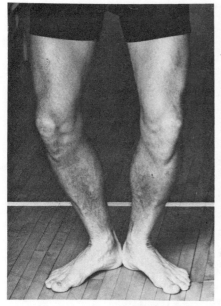
TOES OUT/KNEES OUT

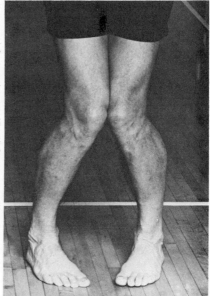
TOES IN/KNEES IN

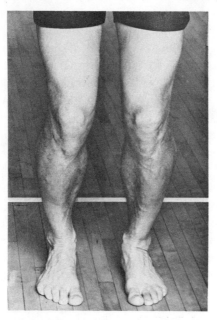
PROPER FOOT PLACEMENT

Fallen Arches and Pronating Heels

If you look back at the illustration of the foot and its multiple interconnecting arches, you are reminded that this handsome-looking arch is held in suspension by ligaments and muscles. That's the way the foot should be built, but a great many people are born with very little arch or what we call fallen arches or flat feet. Many others lose their arch support with normal aging.

People with fallen arches eventually develop a turning in, or pronation, of the ankles. The easiest way to recognize pronation is to stand barefoot and have someone sight down your Achilles tendon. If the tendons follow a straight line through the ankle to the heel, you are okay. If, instead, the tendons bend inward, as in the illustration on page 199, your problem is simple pronation.

Pronation of the ankles is a very common cause of pain in the feet, legs, and knees. Some athletes try to put up with the discomfort as part of the game as long as the pain isn't crippling, but this is not necessary, as one weekend athlete discovered.

A middle-aged West Point officer recalls developing Achilles tendinitis in both legs and occasional pain in his right knee. When he got up in the morning, both Achilles tendons hurt until he warmed up with stretching exercises or hobbled around for a few minutes. But that didn't help for long. If he sat still for more than fifteen minutes, the tendons would bother him again. Standing was painful, and he then had to walk stiff-legged until the tendons warmed up. This went on for about two years.

The man thought that he was paying a price for playing hard at handball, racquetball, squash, tennis, and basketball, that these pains had to be accepted as "overuse" pains—the price of continuing to play hard in the middle years. Then one day, after creaking out of the shower, he noticed that when he put weight on his feet, there was a pronounced turning in of his ankles. He looked at his feet carefully in a mirror, and sure enough, they were pronating.

This weekender was lucky. He remembered a lecture at West Point by Professor Karl K. Klein of the University of Texas Rehabilitation Laboratory, a consultant to the Department of Physical Education at West Point, who is one of the nation's top exercise physiologists. The weekender bought a pair of foot supports that

NORMAL HEEL AND PRONATING HEEL

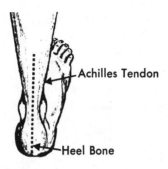

NORMAL HEEL

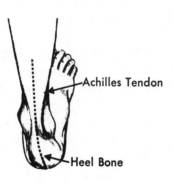

PRONATING HEEL

Professor Klein had recommended, and his problems disappeared. He also began using felt arch supports in his tennis, basketball, and running shoes. Since then, he has pain in his tendons and knees only if he plays without the supports.

The Ankle

The ankle is one of the most complicated joints of the body. It is a sort of hinge connecting the talus bone of the foot to the bottom surfaces of the two lower leg bones—the tibia and the fibula—with all three held together by a maze of ligaments, tendons, and muscles. The most common ankle injury is a sprain, which is a partial tear of the ligament tissue.*

The site of a sprain is usually at one of two major groups of ligaments:

• LCL, the lateral (or external) collateral ligament, which is on the outside of the ankle.

• MCL, the medial collateral ligament, which is on the inside of the ankle.

The LCL, a three-branch ligament, is the one commonly injured. This occurs when a person lands on the outer edge of the ankle, rolls over it, and thus "twists" the ankle. The LCL branch normally affected by the roll-over is the anterior talofibular (see illustration, page 201).

The MCL is a fan-shaped ligament which prevents the foot from turning outward excessively. It is normally very strong and effective. However, when the ligaments are loose, ankles are accordingly weak.

Sprains are best treated by rest until the pain disappears, followed by reconditioning exercises to help strengthen the muscles of the lower leg and foot in order to increase support of the ankle.

A tendency to turn your ankle or any other signals of ankle weakness should have prompt attention. The more often the ligament is damaged, the less effectively it stabilizes the ankle, and the less stabilized the ankle, the more often you damage the ligament. It's

---

* Some laymen are never certain about the difference between a strain and a sprain. A sprain is a tear of the ligament fibrous tissue, usually in and around the joint. A strain is a tear of the fibrous tissue of the muscle-tendon complex.

THE ANKLE

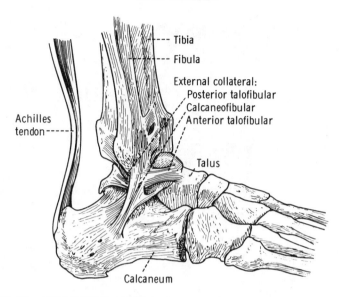

LATERAL (OUTSIDE) VIEW OF THE ANKLE SHOWING THE THREE BRANCHES OF THE EXTERNAL (LATERAL) COLLATERAL LIGAMENT

a bad cycle that should be terminated with specific conditioning. The exercises previously described under "Movements of the Foot" (page 188) should be used to strengthen the muscles of the lower leg and foot in order to help the ligaments support the ankle.

The ankle is the most vulnerable major joint in the body, the most likely to be sprained. High-top shoes and ankle wraps can help to give support. The most vulnerable area in the lower leg is the Achilles tendon, the most likely to be strained.

The Achilles Tendon

The bones that run from the ankle to the knee are called the tibia and the fibula. The major calf muscles are called the gastrocnemius and the soleus. Both groups of muscles share a common tendon, the Achilles, which attaches to the heel bone, the calcaneus. The Achilles is the thickest and strongest tendon in the whole body. It has to be, and you should know why.

THE ACHILLES TENDON

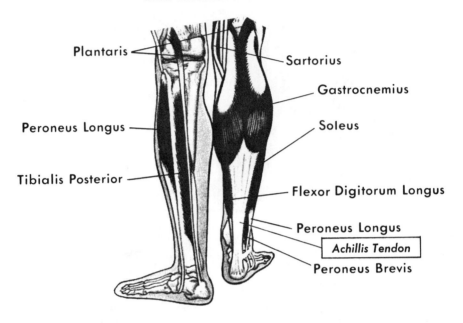

Plantaris

Peroneus Longus

Tibialis Posterior

Sartorius

Gastrocnemius

Soleus

Flexor Digitorum Longus

Peroneus Longus

Achillis Tendon

Peroneus Brevis

If you check the illustration on page 201, you see that the entire weight of the body rides down the tibia and fibula and rests on the talus bone. The talus bone then rides on the top front of the calcaneus and thus requires a very strong stabilizer to maintain the body's balance and propel the body from one foot to the other. The Achilles tendon is the rope by which the calf muscles, when contracting, raise the weight of the body that is concentrated on one foot and, by raising, shifts the weight-bearing responsibility to the other foot.

Achilles tendonitis is common with runners, skiers, tennis players, or any athlete who must run, jump, turn, or change direction rapidly.

Tendon strain may be caused by some of the foot problems already noted or underconditioning of calf muscles and the Achilles tendons. When the Achilles tendons are too tight, they are more susceptible to tearing, and this is the reason flexibility is emphasized. To determine if the tendons are too tight, try walking on your heels while barefoot. If you cannot, you have tendons that are too tight.

To maintain flexibility, the Achilles tendons must be stretched in a controlled manner because they are not basically elastic. It takes patience and time to do this. Don't expect overnight results. Go about it gradually and continuously. Remember, if you stop stretching, you will lose flexibility again.

Two excellent exercises for increasing flexibility in the Achilles tendon are:

1. *Heel Dip* (see page 204). This may be done on a stairway or thick big book. Stairs would be better. While holding onto the rail with one hand, place the balls of your feet on the edge of a step (or book) with the remainder of your feet unsupported. Slowly drop your heels below the level of your toes until you feel your Achilles tendon stretch behind your heel. Hold the position for 15 seconds at first, and over a period of 14 to 21 days increase to 45 seconds. Repeat the exercise 2 or 3 times a day if you are very inflexible. *Caution*: Do not bounce while stretching!

2. *Achilles Stretch.* See Exercise 1 under "Flexibility," page 98.

Shin Splints/Stress Fractures

Shin splints are the bane of the out-of-condition and beginning athlete. The splints are generally recognized as tiny tears in the anterior tibial muscles at the point of insertion into the tibia, the shin. These muscles, which extend along the front of the bone from the knee to the foot, move the foot and toes. The injury known as shin splints is usually caused by overexertion, running strenuously on hard surfaces, improper foot placement, pronation, or overweight —even as little as five pounds.

Stress fractures (see page 205) are not really fractures or breaks as we know them, but the bone's reaction to fatigue when it is subject to more intense and repeated stress than the tibia has been conditioned to handle. Bones, like muscles, can be conditioned through small and gradual amounts of stress to become stronger. However, when there is too much stress, especially if the stress is persistent and intense, the bone "fails" before it is able to adapt to the greater demand.

It is difficult for the physician to distinguish between shin splints and stress fracture. Typically an athlete may receive a diagnosis of shin splints only to have the diagnosis changed to stress fracture some three weeks later when the X ray first shows the shadow of

HEEL DIP EXERCISE

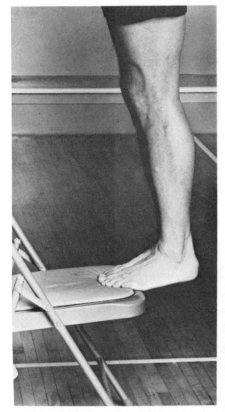

STARTING POSITION

STRETCH POSITION—HOLD

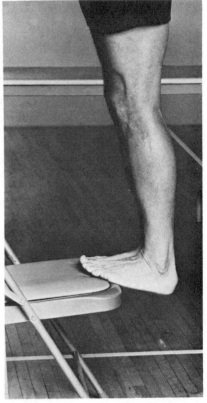

STRESS FRACTURES

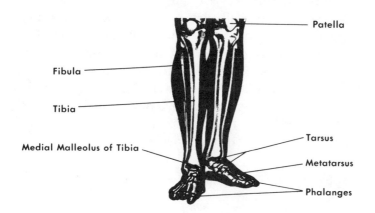

Patella

Fibula

Tibia

Medial Malleolus of Tibia

Tarsus

Metatarsus

Phalanges

1. FRONT SKELETAL VIEW

THE TIBIA AND THE METATARSALS ARE THE MOST
COMMON SITES FOR STRESS FRACTURES.

new bone which finally distinguishes clearly between the two injuries.

Normally the pain from a stress fracture localizes on a relatively small area of the bone, while shin splints hurt the length of the tibia. Less frequently the metatarsal bones of the foot may suffer stress fractures.

At West Point we find that women cadets are more commonly injured by shin splints and stress fractures than the men by a ratio of about 10 to 1. This can't be explained by any physiological difference, and we believe that it reflects a cultural difference: that most women are not as well conditioned as the men when they first arrive at the Academy. In fact, the best prevention of shin splints and stress fracture is to intensify workouts more gradually and progressively. Other ways of preventing these injuries include weight reduction, proper foot placement, and shoes that cushion the feet against hard surfaces.

The treatment for both injuries includes reduced activity and perhaps complete rest for the leg, especially in the event of stress fracture.

The Knee

Just as gladiators gave the ancient physician Galen the opportunity to study anatomy, football players have advanced the practice of knee surgery. The Namath Knee has come to be part of the heraldry of the gridiron. We don't merely have an occasional knee injury; we have an epidemic of knee injuries. Sometimes it seems to good ole coach that everyone on the field has a knee ailment except the pompon girls. But ole coach is wrong. Pompon girls hurt their knees, too. In fact, most knee injuries occur in nonviolent sports, including tennis, swimming, golf, and bowling.

FRONT VIEW OF RIGHT KNEE, 1

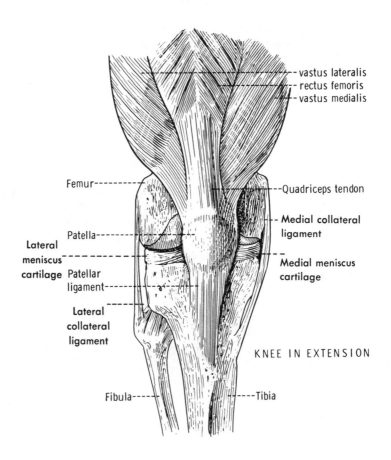

vastus lateralis
rectus femoris
vastus medialis

Femur

Quadriceps tendon

Medial collateral ligament

Patella

Lateral meniscus cartilage

Patellar ligament

Medial meniscus cartilage

Lateral collateral ligament

KNEE IN EXTENSION

Fibula

Tibia

The knee appears to be a simple hinge, yet it is a constant challenge and puzzle. Sports medicine physicians attend conferences to exchange notes on how to treat various knee injuries. They talk about "conservative" methods, which mean therapy without operating—and then they discuss the newest surgical techniques. They talk for hours, and some think the knees may be the most important joint of the body. Certainly, it is the most complicated.

The knee joint is formed by the top surface of the shinbone (tibia) and the bottom surface of the upper leg, the thighbone (femur). It is at the knee that the weight-bearing bones of the leg meet and articulate. However, the bone surfaces never come into direct contact. Sandwiched between the bones are the lateral and the medial meniscus cartilages. These cartilages are attached to the bones and represent the primary cushions in absorbing the body's weight. These spongy cushions also secrete a lubricating fluid which further reduces friction when the bones move.

The third bone called the patella, better known as the kneecap, functions in a remarkable way. It acts like a pulley and provides a

FRONT VIEW OF RIGHT KNEE, 2

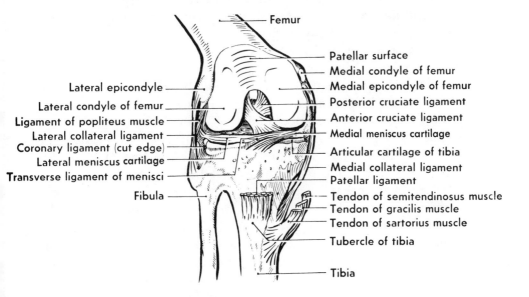

Note: Patella is removed to show interior ligaments

better angle for the front upper-leg muscles (the quadriceps) to lift with greater strength and efficiency. The patella "floats" in front of the ends of the femur and tibia, nesting on the networks of two separate fiber bundles, the tendon fibers of the quadriceps muscles and the fibers of its own patellar ligament.

The stability of the knee hinge is vital. It depends on two sets of ligaments—the collaterals and the cruciates. The collaterals pass along the inside and the outside of the joint, working in concert to stabilize the knee and prevent its moving from side to side.

The short, thick cruciate ligaments attach diagonally inside the knee to the converging bone surfaces, forming an X. The cruciates stabilize the forward and backward movement of the knee hinge.

The muscles and tendons are secondary stabilizers but very important because they help protect the ligaments from shock. If the upper-leg muscles, the quadriceps, or the hamstrings are weak, the knee is that much more susceptible to injury.

Please understand that the preceding is an oversimplification of a very complex network of muscles, tendons, ligaments, bones, and nerves.

There are all kinds of popular names for knee injuries, including jumper's knee, dancer's knee, surfer's knee, and housemaid's knee. Weekend athletes often talk of a trick knee, which may suddenly give way or, as suddenly, lock without warning. This may occur during a game, when you are walking stairways, or if you are merely crossing your legs.

Most such knee malfunctions are usually the result of incompletely treated or unattended prior injuries which consequently cause instability in the knee joint. For example, a common cause of knee injury is a blow to the knee that stretches the medial collateral ligament and may also pull or tear the medial meniscus cartilage to which the medial collateral ligament attaches.

When ligaments are damaged, they can be repaired only through surgery. However, the muscles can be strengthened in their role as stabilizer, and this has proved very effective in West Point's rehabilitation program, a model recommended by sports medicine experts. One division of the rehabilitation program is the Knee Squad, which has become famous in sports circles. Out of this research we have learned that if muscles of both legs are not equally strong, the weaker leg is more likely to incur a knee injury. Consequently each new class of cadets is surveyed for any past knee injuries or problems.

We insist that cadets report any prior knee injuries no matter how minor because we know from our research that most hurt knees result in the problem leg's becoming weaker and the "good" leg's being favored and becoming stronger. So we compare the strength of the hamstrings and quadriceps of each leg. If there is more than a 10 percent differential of bilateral strength between the muscle groups of the two legs, the cadet is assigned to the Knee Squad and put on an exercise routine to strengthen the muscles of both legs. The exercises continue until the bilateral strength differential is less than 10 percent. Because both legs are strengthened, the affected leg normally ends up stronger than the "good" leg was before beginning the program.

The research has taught us to avoid certain rehabilitative exercises such as deep knee bends, squat jumps, and duck walks because these tend to stretch the cruciate ligaments and thus weaken the inner stability of the knee. Instead, we concentrate on strengthening the thigh muscles—the quadriceps in the front and hamstrings in the back as a means of stabilizing the knee joint. The best method of doing this is to use special exercise machines such as the Orthotron/Cybex. However, these are normally available only in rehabilitation centers or research offices. Calisthenic exercises to help stabilize the knee joint are part of each of the GAF levels, e.g., Half Squat in Level I (page 132), Squat Thrust in Level II (page 149), and Step-ups in Level III (page 166). In addition, the quadriceps and hamstring flexibility exercises are part of the flexibility series (see Part III).

The Thighs

If you glance back at the skeletal illustrations (pages 181 and 182), you'll see they are not just pictures devised to organize this material for you. In a real sense, they describe the way that the body "grows" upward from the fifty-two bones of the feet through the four bones of the calves to the heavy two bones of the thighs. Reverse direction, and you see that the upper body mass, for the first time, divides its weight load to pass through the two femurs, fanning progressively downward through the calves and the feet in an intricate concert of load-bearing distribution and mobility.

As noted in the description of the knee, the lower end of the femur helps form the knee. The top end of the femur angles inward in a ball-like shape to ride inside the pelvic socket and thus forms the hip, the joint that connects the upper and lower body. The hip is mainly dependent on muscles to function properly. The muscles most commonly injured by physical activity are the quadriceps and hamstrings, which lift and pull back the legs, and the inner groin muscles, which hold the legs in center position and also return the legs to that position when spread.

The most common injury in the thigh area is muscle strain, such as a hamstring pull, and this is caused by muscular imbalance. As noted earlier, skeletal muscles work in antagonistic pairs. For instance, the hamstrings and quadriceps are antagonistic pairs. When you run, the quadriceps raise and flex the knees while the hamstrings lower the knees and brake the accelerated force. When one group of antagonistic muscles is considerably stronger than the other one, you are likely to have an injury.

The hamstrings work with gravity while quadriceps work against gravity. Therefore, the quadriceps are usually stronger. Research finds that the differential range between the strength of the two muscles generally is as much as 50 percent. However, when the quadriceps are more than 50 percent stronger than the hamstrings, the two muscle groups are considered in a state of imbalance. In a sports event when the stronger muscle group can overpower the weaker, such as a sprint or a sharp cut while you play basketball, handball, or tennis, the possibility of a pulled hamstring is increased significantly.

The general treatment for muscle imbalance is to strengthen the weaker muscles and stretch the stronger one. However, the hamstring must be both strengthened and stretched to prevent hamstring strain. The reason is this: During the running cycle, when the hamstring muscle contracts, it straightens the hip joint at the same time that it bends the knee joint. At the point in the cycle when the knee joint straightens and the hip joint bends, the hamstrings are stretched. This stretching may cause the muscles to tear.

Once you have a hamstring pull, it is a long, slow process to get back to normal again, and this is the best reason to consider stretching and strengthening the hamstrings before the injury

KLEIN'S FLEXIBILITY TEST FOR HAMSTRINGS

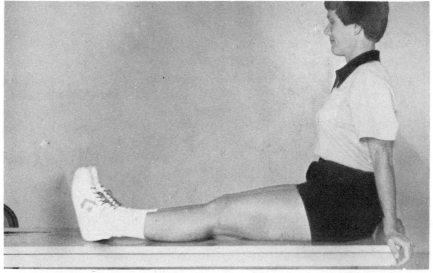

1. SITTING ON TABLE, AS SHOWN ABOVE, SUPPORT TRUNK WITH HANDS, SIT UP STRAIGHT, AND ARCH THE LUMBAR SPINE. IF THE LOWER BACK CANNOT ARCH AND THE LUMBAR CURVE IS ROUNDED, AS IN PICTURE 2, THE HAMSTRINGS ARE TOO TIGHT

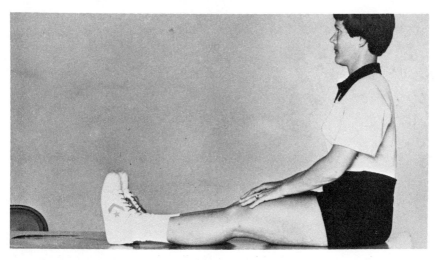

2. NOTE: THE PELVIS IS TIPPED BACKWARD, PREVENTING THE LUMBAR SPINE FROM ARCHING.

occurs. Exercises to prevent hamstring pulls are included in the GAF flexibility section. These are specifically GAF Flexibility Exercises 2, 3, and 4 (pages 100–105). Remember, the hamstring pull is considered a preventable injury in 99 percent of the cases. It is generally an indication of an inadequate or poor conditioning program.

Groin Pulls

Groin pull is usually caused by the forced spreading of the legs that may happen when a person slips. The muscles strained are called adductors, high up on the inner sides of the thighs. The adductors make the attachment between the interior of the hip to the inner surface of the femur and thereby control sideward movement of the legs.

You can develop flexibility of the groin muscles with a simple exercise called the Groin Stretch. (See Exercise 6 in GAF flexibility series, page 108).

Chapter 14

The Upper Body and Its Best Parts

The upper body rides on the two ball-like tops of the femurs that fit like bearings into the sockets of the hip.

The spine is a movable column, the supporting axis for the entire body. The spine is continuously involved with intermeshing forces, constantly bending, twisting, and extending itself.

The head rides at the summit of this column, turning, lifting, twitching, continuously articulating, constantly responding to the environment.

The organs, including the heart, lungs, kidneys, liver, and intestines, in the upper body are vital.

The bones, ligaments, and muscles protect and defend the life support system.

The upper body is usable in bruising, contact sports as well as in developing delicate skills and agility.

In fact, the upper body thrives on use.

Taking it from the top, reversing direction, we pass down through the seven vertebrae of the neck to the rib cage and upper back.

The scapulae (shoulder blades) are winglike bones which lie atop the sides of the upper back. They contain the sockets for the bones of the upper arms. Together, they form the shoulder joints.

The clavicles (collarbones) attach at the base of the neck to the sternum, like a horizontal bar, across and over the rib cage, stiff-arming, as it were, the scapulae in place. This whole mechanism is the shoulder girdle from which the shoulder joints move the arms, attached and yet free of the torso (see illustration on page 214).

The sternum (breastbone) is a tough cartilage strip down the center of the upper chest. The sternum grips the ribs as they curve around the spine and gives an additional degree of elasticity to the cage structure.

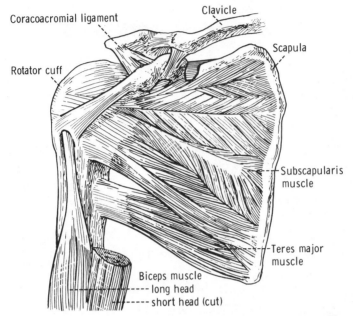

Coracoacromial ligament

Clavicle

Rotator cuff

Scapula

Subscapularis muscle

Teres major muscle

Biceps muscle
----- long head
----- short head (cut)

FRONT VIEW—RIGHT SHOULDER

REAR VIEW—RIGHT SHOULDER

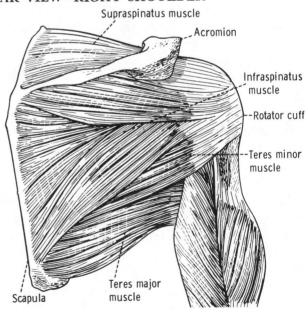

Supraspinatus muscle

Acromion

Infraspinatus muscle

Rotator cuff

Teres minor muscle

Scapula

Teres major muscle

High under the rib cage are the vital systems of the lungs and heart. With the descending mound of other soft organs, they are bound in place behind thick bandages of back and abdominal ligaments, muscles, and tendons, which wall the gap between the cavity of the rib cage and the hollow of the pelvic girdle.

Earlier we described the body weight as being distributed like a fan through the legs and feet which helps achieve agility in the lower body parts. A like process of fanning occurs in the upper arms, elbows, lower arms, wrists, and hands, the sum of which accounts for dexterity in these parts of the upper body.

The Back

The spine supports the weight of the upper body, absorbs shock, and provides for a wide range of torso movements. This is possible because the vertebral column is flexible, composed of twenty-four separate vertebrae plus the sacrum (tailbone) and coccyx. The twenty-four vertebrae include the seven of the neck plus twelve thoracic (upper-back) vertebrae and five lumbar (lower-back) vertebrae.

The spinal cord is rarely involved in ordinary kinds of sports injury. Although the supporting muscle and ligament in the neck are reduced in order to allow flexibility of the head, the upper-back and lower-back regions of the spinal cord are stabilized with strong supporting musculature.

Sports, such as diving and acrobatics, which place the neck region in the most stress are normally controlled by the training and ability of the performer. However, sports research finds that in contact sports the incident of neck injury has increased and directly correlates with the increased use of head and face protective gear. Researchers guess that headgear gives the athlete a false sense of security. As a result, normal caution and awareness of risk are thrown to the winds. The player gets involved in greater levels of force than he should and literally puts his neck on the line. For those athletes, strengthening of the neck muscles is essential. Fortunately, however, the weekender does not use the head as a weapon, and few neck injuries are attributed to weekend sports activities. The stiff neck comes from the player's suddenly twisting the head in serving in tennis before he warms up properly. Although this is a troublesome injury, it is not serious. It can be prevented by his rolling the head in a circle, both clockwise and counterclockwise, as part of the precompetition workout. It is safe to say that we seldom see the weekender in a neck brace. Most of the weekender's problems are from pain in the lower back.

Low-Back Pain

A major problem in low-back pain is the reaction of the athlete. The weekender is inclined to resign himself to an inactive life, and that will make his back worse. The professional athlete is likely to mask the suffering with a pain-killer, which again does nothing to resolve the problem, and that's too bad. There's no mystery about low-back pain. Usually it's a muscular problem that can be corrected in your own home, often rather easily.

Although the back is a complicated network of bones, cartilage, ligaments, nerves, blood vessels, and muscles, most low-back pain is the result of abnormal stretching of the ligaments of the spine. This is caused by muscular imbalance which pulls the body out of shape. When some muscles are strong, others weak, and there is a lack of flexibility, one hip may be high, the other low, the pelvis tilts, and the spine curves too much.

These are not congenital defects but simply a result of poor sitting, standing, and walking habits. These posture problems may be subtle, unnoticeable when a person is clothed, but they are so common that every cadet who enters West Point is examined for these faults. You have to get beneath the clothing and below the skin to understand what's going on.

As a starter, you should understand that the whole weight of the body is concentrated in the lumbar region of the lower back. To compensate for this, the lumbar vertebrae are broader and heavier than the vertebrae in the upper back and neck. The muscles of the back, abdomen, and hips attach to the lumbar vertebrae, and these muscles have to be brought into balance to eliminate back pain.

There are several muscle groups that act as guy wires to support and move the spine. One group, the extensors, has the primary function of arching the back, bending it backward, and holding the back stiff and erect. The extensors are a mixed, complicated set of multi-layered short and long muscles.

Another group, the lateral muscles, controls side bending. The lateral group includes the psoas major, one of the largest single muscles in the body. The psoas major attaches to the lumbar vertebrae and passes through the pelvis to the top surface of the thighbone just below the hip joint. It has been called a two-joint muscle because it controls not only the back but also the hips and legs. The psoas major is a short, powerful muscle and a troublemaker. The psoas major is most subject to stress which results in pain, and the persons most susceptible are the soft-bellied.

One of the best ways to counteract overloading of the psoas major is to strengthen the abdominal muscle group, which is anchored to the rib cage. Besides supporting the abdomen, these muscles extend to the side and front of the pelvis. When the abdominals are strong, they go to work for you, preventing low-back pain by pulling up the front of the pelvis, giving your stomach good support, and flattening excessive curvature in your back. The best exercises for strengthening the abdominals are the Bent-Knee Curl (1) and the Bent-Knee Sit-up (2). See these exercises in the GAF section: (1), page 143, and (2), page 160.

Other muscles involved in low-back pain are the muscles of the hip. These include four groups that have the responsibility for hip abduction—(spreading the legs), hip adduction (closing the legs), hip flexion (raising the legs), and hip extension (bringing them back). These are very complicated muscle groups, but in some dancing circles they are known simply as the bumps and grinds.

One of the most important hip extensors is the gluteus maximus, also known as the butt muscle, the muscle that forms a bun when you tighten your buttocks. Sprinters have highly developed gluteus maximus muscles because they are the primary source of running power. The gluteus muscles and the other hip extensors, such as the hamstrings, help control pelvis tilt and swayback.

When muscle imbalance occurs, the hip flexors are tight, and the abdominals and hip extensors weak. The pelvis tilts forward, causing an excess curve or sway in the area of the lumbar vertebrae or low back. This swayback curve causes the lumbar vertebrae to bend forward, and the back sides of the vertebrae are forced closer together (pinched). This presses on the nerves, and the pressure causes pain and muscle spasm in the low back. The forward pelvis tilt also causes overstretching of the hamstrings, which may cause

KLEIN'S FLEXIBILITY TEST FOR PSOAS

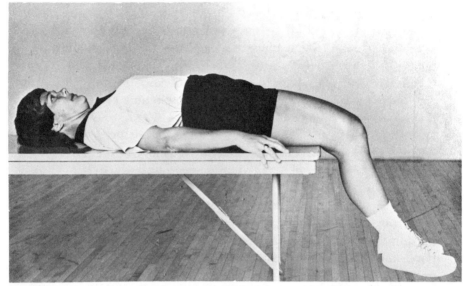

1. LIE WITH BACK ON TABLE; ALLOW THE LOWER LEGS TO HANG OVER THE EDGE. PULL ONE KNEE TO THE CHEST.

2. IF THE OPPOSITE LEG RISES OFF THE TABLE, THE PSOAS IS TOO TIGHT ON THAT SIDE.

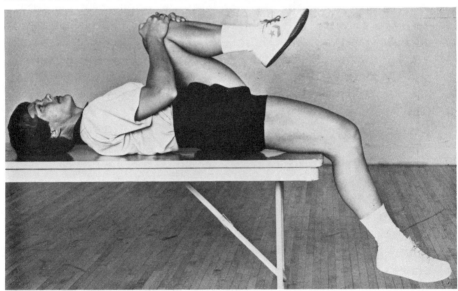

early hamstring fatigue and hamstring pull. Functionally the forward pelvis tilt will result in a shorter stride for a distance runner.

Acute and prolonged cases of muscle imbalance may result in severe problems such as slipped disk, especially in the lumbar region. A slipped disk is actually degeneration of a joint between the vertebrae. If it is allowed to reach an advanced stage, prolonged treatment or even surgery may be necessary.

Slipped disk is not a sudden occurrence. Disk degeneration is gradual after many warnings from episodes with low-back pain. That is why back pain should be taken seriously. The following exercises, chosen by Professor Klein for the cadets, are designed to prevent low back pain by increasing muscular flexibility and strength:

LOW BACK EXERCISES
(PARTIAL WILLIAMS SERIES)

EXERCISE 1. BENT-KNEE CURL

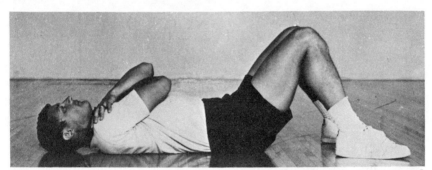

STARTING POSITION

HOLD POSITION

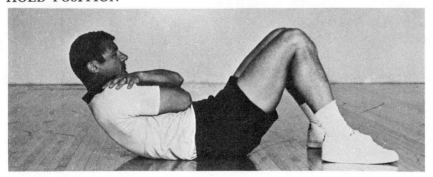

EXERCISE 2. PELVIC FLATTENER

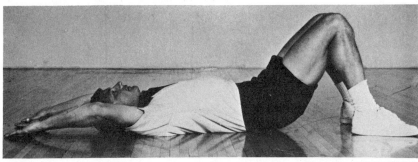

HOLD POSITION

EXERCISE 3. BACK STRETCHER

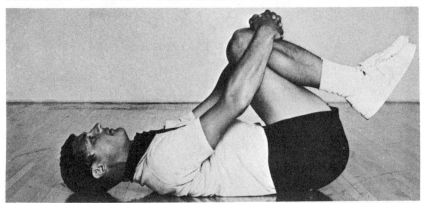

STARTING POSITION

HOLD POSITION

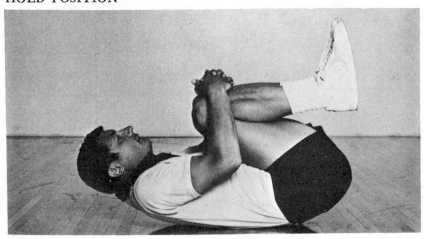

EXERCISE 4. PSOAS STRETCHER

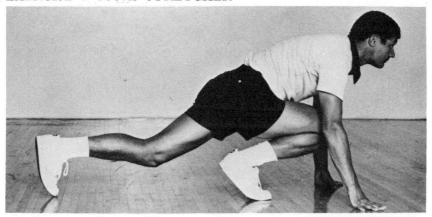

HOLD POSITION

EXERCISE 5. HAMSTRING STRETCH

STARTING POSITION

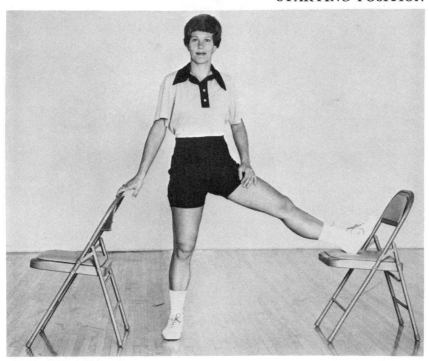

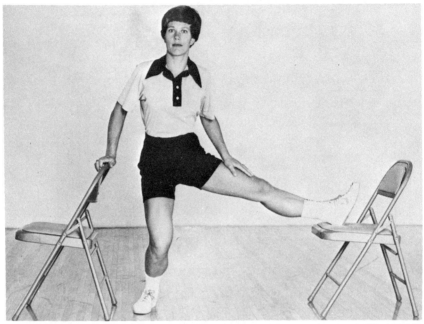

HOLD POSITION

EXERCISE 6. TRUNK ROTATOR STRETCH

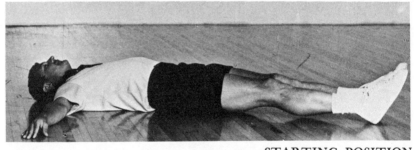

STARTING POSITION

HOLD POSITION

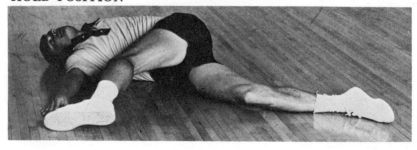

EXERCISE 7. ACHILLES STRETCH

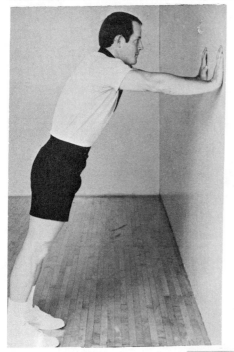

STARTING POSITION

ACTION-HOLD POSITION

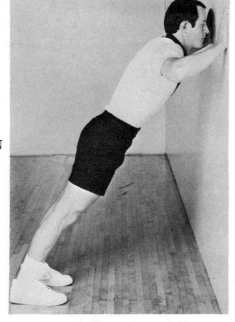

EXERCISE 8. RECTUS FEMORIS STRETCH

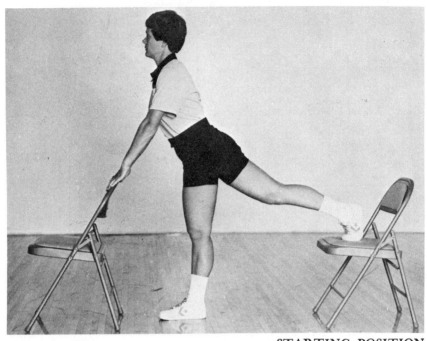

STARTING POSITION

HOLD POSITION

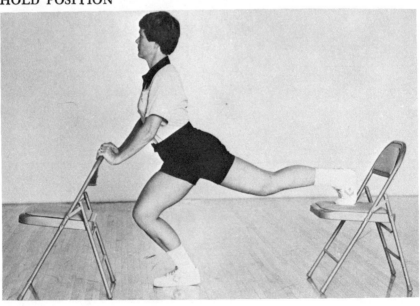

The Arm and the Shoulder

Most injuries to the hand and wrist are accidents: A bad fall sprains the wrist or dislocates the small joints of the fingers; a ball causes hyperextension of the fingers, spreading and spraining the fingers or thumb; or the hand is cut as you open a can of tennis balls. Since these are accidental, they aren't preventable by exercise. The only thing to do is get off into a corner and curse your bad luck, and then remember that such accidents happen to all of us some of the time.

On the other hand, the common and chronic complaints about shoulders—tennis shoulder, thrower's shoulder, bowler's shoulder, etc.—and elbows—tennis elbow, golfer's elbow, handball elbow, etc. —are usually due to tendinitis but tendinitis is an effect, not a cause. Once you know the cause, you can do something about it, and you should do so quickly, and then all the elbows and thrower's shoulders will live happily ever after.

The shoulder joint, one of the largest in the body, is formed by the humerus (the upper arm) and the scapula (shoulder blade). A ball-shaped projection of the humerus moves inside the socket of the scapula, allowing for a wide range of motions. The muscles and tendons of the shoulder hold these two bones in place and stabilize the shoulder through the full range of motion (see illustration on page 214).

Of the many groups of muscles in the shoulders, the ones that most concern the weekend athlete are the deltoids, which raise the shoulder and arm; the biceps, which flex and move the shoulder and arm; and the rotator cuff, a group of four muscles, three of which rotate the shoulder outward and a fourth which turns it inward. Some of the athletic activities that require the combined use of all these muscles are swimming, tennis, handball, bowling, skiing, golf, and any throwing action. However, it is the tendons, the tough inelastic tissues that attach muscles to bones, that suffer the most and pass along the pain.

The most common shoulder tendinitis occurs at two points: where the biceps muscle tendon attaches to the scapula and where the tendon of the rotator cuff muscles attaches to the humerus. Biceps tendinitis is caused by a lack of conditioning, perhaps when you return to a seasonal sport and begin to throw too hard or in cross-country skiing where powerful poling motions are required.

Tendon inflammation also results when you serve a ball incorrectly in tennis or when you throw while off-balance. This may happen even to a pro who decides to play hurt. The most famous instance was the case of the great Dizzy Dean, the St. Louis Cardinal pitcher, who broke his toe but continued pitching. Dean changed his style of delivery to compensate for the painful toe and wound up wrecking his pitching arm permanently. But for most of us, especially weekend athletes, the problem is a lack of fitness, the preparation for physical activity. As with any tendon injury, resting the affected body part is necessary to the healing process. To prevent strain, conditioning exercises for the shoulder are to be found in Part II, "GAF." Stretching as well as strengthening exercises are important.

The Elbow and Lower Arm

The elbow is a hinge joint formed by three bones: the humerus (the bone of the upper arm) and the larger ulna and the thinner, lighter radius (the two bones of the lower arm). The radius curves in such a way as to form the lower, inner part of the elbow joint and the outer part of the wrist joint on the little-finger side of the

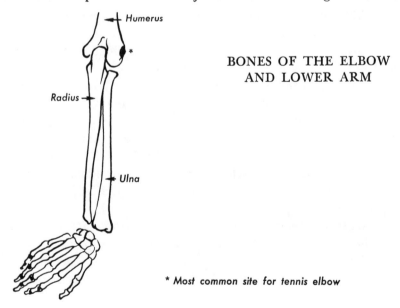

BONES OF THE ELBOW
AND LOWER ARM

* Most common site for tennis elbow

hand. Conversely, the ulna curves to the thumb side of the hand and the outside part of the elbow joint. It is this naturally designed torque that allows the wrist to rotate and move outward and inward in relation to the elbow, which is solely a hinge joint.

Until joggers began beating up their Achilles tendon, tennis elbow was the most talked-about ailment of the weekend athlete. Now that it ranks second, tennis elbow is just as painful. The sensation is something like having a sewing machine jabbing at the outside of the elbow if the problem is your backhand, the inside edge if it's your forehand (see illustration on page 228).

Doctors have prescribed cortisone shots, aspirin and other anti-inflammatory medication, hot packs or cold packs—dry and wet—and rest. When the weekender picked up a racquet again, the sewing machine continued etching in the pain because doctors were treating symptoms, not the cause, which is insufficient muscle conditioning. Most weekend athletes suffer from backhand tennis elbows caused by underconditioned forearm muscles or hitting the backhand incorrectly.

The backhand stroke stresses the muscles that straighten or extend the wrist. This requires strong and well-developed extensor muscles (see the illustration on page 228). These muscles seldom get an adequate workout, such as lifting, in normal day-to-day activity.

There are three groups of extensor muscles that are stressed in the backhand stroke: the carpi ulnaris, the carpi radial brevis, and the digitorum communis. All three groups have their origin on the outside (lateral) condyle of the upper-arm bone.

The lateral and the medial (inside) condyles of the upper-arm bone are the two bony bumps on either side of the elbow joint. To locate these easily, feel the joint when the palm is face up. The flexor muscle groups of the wrist begin at the medial condyle and are the ones most commonly used in daily activity, such as picking up small objects, playing the piano, or throwing.

Also attached to the medial condyle are two other muscle groups related to tennis elbow—the pronators, which turn the palm down, and the supinators, which turn the palm up. Repeated pronation when you hit forehand strokes or a hard-sliced serve and follow through on the same side of the body instead of across the body are major causes of tennis elbow at the medial condyle.

Another cause of stress on the condyle attachment sites is a weak

ELBOW JOINT (TENNIS ELBOW)

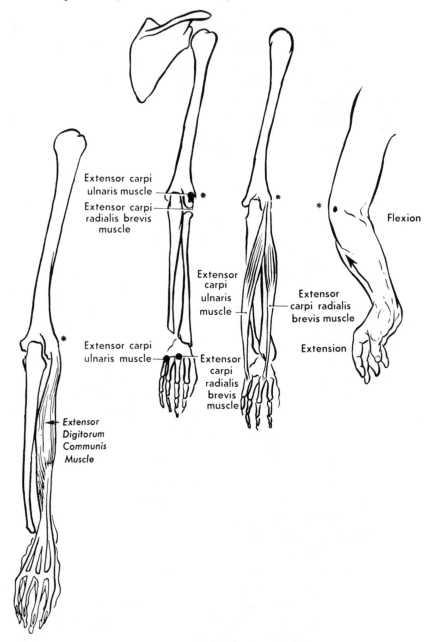

Extensor carpi
ulnaris muscle

Extensor carpi
radialis brevis
muscle

Extensor
carpi
ulnaris
muscle

Extensor
carpi radialis
brevis muscle

Flexion

Extension

Extensor carpi
ulnaris muscle

Extensor
carpi
radialis
brevis
muscle

Extensor
Digitorum
Communis
Muscle

• Sites of muscle attachment   * Most common site for tennis elbow grip, also a factor in off-center hits. Similarly, a whipping action in the wrist when you try to put top spin on the ball may damage the elbow as well as the hand, wrist, and forearm muscles.

Proper stroking technique is one key to the prevention of tennis elbow, and a visit to your tennis pro for an analysis of your form is advisable.

Equipment is important. The racquet should not be too tightly strung. The grip should be correct. A small grip forces you to squeeze the racquet too much in order to prevent its turning in your hand, and an oversize grip creates difficulty in controlling strokes. Both these problems add stress to the elbow.

Still, at the base of good technique itself are flexibility and strength. You'll find the required conditioning exercises in Parts II and IV that will take you far toward preventing tennis elbow.

Two reminders: Going from one sport to another without specific conditioning may result in twinges of tennis elbow. For example, many weekend athletes play tennis during the spring and summer and then play other games, such as squash, in the fall and winter. However, when you go from a squash to a tennis racquet without conditioning, you are increasing the weight that your hand must bear, and it's enough of an increase to irritate the tendons.

The other reminder is for those who are twenty-year veterans of the weekend tennis court. Unfortunately the mature player is likely to experience tennis elbow after going through most of his life without feeling a twinge. This can be explained and prevented.

To begin with, the time most weekenders put into playing tennis is not enough by itself to maintain adequate strength, much less to develop strong muscles. Furthermore, as the years go by, the muscles naturally get weaker, not stronger. Thus, the combination of normal aging and an absence of conditioning takes its toll. However, a moderate conditioning program will prevent strength loss and tennis elbow.

Remember that pills deal with pain. Conditioning, technique, and proper equipment will prevent tennis elbow.

Safeguarding the Eye

The great increase in popularity of racquet sports has brought with it an increase in the number and severity of eye injuries. West

Point cadets are now required to wear eye protectors during class instruction and intramural participation in racquet games. At the same time we have initiated a program to convince all other players of racquet sports to wear eye protectors no matter what their level of play.

Although it may be expected that an experienced player would develop a strategy to avoid injury, studies find that eye accidents have little relationship to the ability of the player. Indeed, the better player has the tendency to play more competitively and hit harder, thereby increasing the risk of injury.

The risk increases in sports that don't require a net, such as squash, handball, racquetball, and paddle ball. When opponents are playing in the same area, the danger is not only from the ball but also from the racquet and the opponent's hand, as in the case of handball.

The threat to your eyes in net games may not be quite so high but is still present. There is always the danger of being hit in the eye by a ball or shuttlecock. In one instance we saw a weekender as he was running to his baseline to return a lob try to hit the ball over his left shoulder. Instead, he hit himself in the eye with his racquet and had to have five stitches in his left eyebrow.

Accidents like this happen, and there is no conditioning that will prevent them. So eye protectors are in order for everyone who plays. If you're part of the 50 percent of the population that wears eyeglasses, your lenses are likely to be shatterproof, as required by law. However, the frames may not be strong enough to retain the lens if struck by a ball or racquet, but such frames are available, as are protective eye guards for those who do not need prescription lens.

Chapter 15

Playing Hurt—Should You? First Aid and Coming Back Strong

At the risk of being redundant, we would like to note again that preventive conditioning is the best means of avoiding injury. Having said that, we should state that over the years no one escapes hurt or injury of some kind playing recreational sports. To the beginning weekend athlete it may not make sense that people play a game that will eventually hurt them and, furthermore, that when these same people heal, they come back to play again. A good competitor never goes into a game expecting to be hurt, but it happens.

More surprising to the novice is learning that it's not pain that worries athletes, but the fact that the injury may keep them out of play. Not only the pro worries about being sidelined, but weekenders with whom we met also talked about becoming edgy when sprains or fractures kept them inactive.

What we would like to do in this chapter is discuss playing hurt —should or shouldn't you?—the kind of pain you should respect, first aid, comeback conditioning, and begin by explaining the difference between chronic and acute injuries.

Chronic injuries normally heal by themselves but require your attention and treatment without medical supervision.

Acute injuries require immediate medical attention and, if neglected, may get worse and hamper any further athletic participation.

These are the general rules that most sports medicine physicians believe identify acute injuries:

1. Any injury accompanied by severe pain or swelling should be considered acute.

2. All joint injuries which result from vigorous activity and are accompanied by sudden pain and swelling while you are playing, or immediately after play, should be examined. These injuries usually occur because of a fall or twist.

231

3. A bone or joint pain that lasts fourteen days or longer should be examined, even though the pain is not so severe that you can't use the body part. Remember that something is causing the pain, and the cause needs to be diagnosed.

4. Any injury that you think is chronic but doesn't heal in three weeks should be examined in order to discover the cause.

5. Any injury that nags at your sense of well-being should be checked. Trying to play when you are concerned about an injury will interfere with concentration, will likely cost you the game, and may cause additional injury. When you try to favor an injured part, the result is muscular imbalance.

6. Joint injuries should always be checked by a sports medicine physician before you take up play again. Joint injuries can become permanent if not properly treated.

First Aid for Athletic Injuries

Three steps are recommended for any chronic or acute injury that is severe enough to interrupt a game or for any localized pain that appears shortly after you finish a game.

1. *Apply ice as soon as possible to the injured site.* Ice decreases internal bleeding by causing the injured minute blood vessels to contract. The less blood and other body fluids that collect at the injured site, the sooner it will heal.

To apply ice, put cubes or chips into a plastic bag. Cover the affected area with a towel to prevent damage to the skin. Then place the ice bag on the towel directly over the injured site. The recommended pattern of ice treatment is forty-five minutes on site, fifteen minutes off site. This allows the skin to rewarm and the blood to recirculate. *For an acute injury,* continue the ice treatment until you reach a physician, as long as forty-eight to seventy-two hours, if necessary. *For chronic injury,* the ice treatment should continue for three hours. Then, if the swelling continues and the pain worsens, see a doctor.

2. *Apply compression to the injured site.* Pressure helps prevent swelling. This is easily accomplished by wrapping the applied ice bag to the injured site. If available, an elastic bandage is preferred. The wrap should be taut enough to compress the local area but not so tight as to cut off all blood supply. If the area begins to feel numb

or the pain increases, unwrap the bandage and rewrap less tightly.

3. *Keep the injured part elevated.* Gravity helps to retard the accumulation of blood at the site of the injury if you raise the body part.

Rest for the injured part is important, but this may range from total immobilization of the injured body part to a reduction of activity. For example, if your shoulder gives you discomfort, not pain, following an injury, you may consider modifying your serve to sidearm or underhand and temporarily give up overheads. However, be extremely cautious about allowing anyone to inject drugs, such as steroids, into the site of the injury so that you may play your full game. Although a drug masks the pain, you may aggravate the injury very seriously. Please remember that other parts of the body can and should be kept in shape while the injured part is healing.

Should You Play Hurt?

We admire the scheduled athlete who plays through a game despite an injury. We admire the film hero with an arrow in his chest, a spear piercing his belly, and a tomahawk wedged in his skull who nevertheless dives into white waters to save the heroine from drowning before he steps up to the bar and orders a light beer. None of this should be put down. It symbolizes the triumph of man's spirit over adversity. Still, everything in its proper context.

There's nothing unusual about a pro athlete's playing hurt. Many of us continue to work when we feel rotten. We continue out of a sense of responsibility. In that context we are doing what has to be done, but playing hurt for the purpose of recreation may be dumb. Basically the weekender shouldn't engage in sports when he feels something more than minor discomfort in a body part. Let's note the reasons.

Pain is a message, your body's way of telling you that something is wrong. Drugging yourself to cover up pain closes the door on the intimate dialogue between you and your body. You are no longer aware of what's happening under your skin.

If you forgo pain-killers, the agony becomes a distraction. Threshold pain interferes with your ability to concentrate and play your best.

Finally, when you play hurt, the body attempts to favor the painful part, to readjust body movements in order to lessen the discomfort of pain. When this happens, some body parts are stressed into movements for which they haven't been conditioned.

We noted the Dizzy Dean disaster earlier, but a similar sequence of events can occur in any active sport. Each sport requires its own athletic skill, and each skill is a series of interrelating movements involving numerous body parts in coordination. When one of the parts fails to synchronize with the others, the others will try to compensate. This happens without conscious effort on our part.

For example, a tennis player who rushes back to play after spraining an ankle may find the service motion modified. If the player is still wary about putting weight on the injured ankle, the adjusted service motion may be further modified, resulting in tennis elbow or tennis shoulder.

Bottom Line Rule

In deference to those weekenders who are desperate to get back into the action, we offer one rule to help you exercise your own judgment: If you've had an injury, don't play or exercise the injured part if pain or discomfort continues while you are at rest; if you have only discomfort when the part is being used, you may gradually return to full activity.

Follow these general rules before returning to your favorite sport:

1. Rest only the injured part. Work on the other parts to maintain a level of overall conditioning.

2. While the injured part is recovering—if there is no longer a cast and the range of movement has returned somewhat, as in a knee injury, for instance—work on your cardiorespiratory conditioning by swimming, or try pedaling on a stationary bicycle.

3. When the pain is gone, begin exercising the injured part slowly, and increase workouts gradually. Listen to your body. If you're pushing too hard, pain will tell you to ease up.

One weekender told of how he dealt with an injury that occurred when he was running from the club parking lot to the tennis courts. He was a little late and was cutting across the grass when his left foot caught on a pipe that extended a few inches off the ground. Instead of merely tripping, his foot was trapped by the pipe for a moment, placing stress on his left leg. Worse luck, he fell onto the concrete walk, slamming hard on his left hip and shoulder. There was a sharp pain on the inside of his thigh, and it was excruciating. He got up and tried to walk. He found that he could move gingerly if he bent his knees moderately. When he sat down on a bench, the pain was fierce. He called off the game.

The next morning he decided to find out how badly he was hurt. He could sit comfortably, but he felt pain in the act of getting up or sitting down, stooping, or squatting or when he put his full weight on the leg. Gently he bent over to touch his toes, keeping his knees straight. No pain, and he continued touching his toes to keep his hamstrings flexible.

He raised his right knee to his chest, and then his left knee. No problem. He continued with that exercise. He felt very sore on his left side, over the hip and shoulder where he had hit the concrete. He tried different arm-stretching exercises, and there was no problem. He had full mobility. The bruises didn't interfere with muscle action in his upper body.

Now he knew that he could do a number of exercises to maintain general conditioning, but when he tried a short run down the hall, that hurt. Out of curiosity, he got on his stationary bicycle and surprisingly found that limited rotation in pedaling produced no discomfort. So he added a cardiorespiratory exercise to his workout. After that he eased himself down to the floor to try push-ups. The left leg wouldn't hold his weight. He gave that up. Instead, he got out some old dumbbells. He had no problem.

Now he knew that he could maintain conditioning in his upper body and most of his lower body. He ran through a whole set of exercises every day and within a week had overcome all his pain. The injury was forgotten, and he was back on the courts. No professional was involved, and there was no need for one.

The weekender used a commonsense approach, and he said that he'd used it before: merely testing out different parts of the body to see which ones were okay and could be kept in condition. There's nothing wrong with the weekender's approach, but for your information we would like to include a sophisticated approach used by professionals at West Point when a cadet's injury is serious.

Comeback Conditioning

Comeback conditioning is what it's all about. At the Academy it's called reconditioning, an apt definition because basically we are talking biomechanics, equipment and function. When an injury happens, the basic philosophy is to follow the athlete through a total program to complete recovery which will prevent deconditioning of the well parts of the body while the injured part receives necessary treatment. The principle in preventing deconditioning is use-disuse. When a body part is not used, it atrophies. When used, the body part remains strong. Although the approach to every injury is the same, reconditioning is specific to the body part that has been hurt. As an example, take a typical acute knee injury that requires surgery.

The West Point rehabilitation team includes an orthopedic surgeon, nurse, physical therapist, athletic trainer, and physical education coach. All must coordinate their skills.

The program begins when the surgeon makes the diagnosis and sets a date for surgery. Immediately the physical therapist steps in and starts the patient on exercises for both the good and injured leg prior to surgery. These are exercises the patient can do in bed if necessary.

On the day of the surgery, when the operation is finished, the therapist has the patient continue with the exercises for both legs.

The nurse supervises the postoperative program to ensure that the surgeon's instructions are followed. During the week to ten days of hospitalization the patient goes through a complete series of leg-strengthening exercises twice a day in physical therapy.

Ligament repairs are routinely put in a cast; cartilage operations are not. Three weeks after surgery if there is no cast, or three weeks after a cast is removed, the cadet begins isokinetic resistance exercises on the Cybex II * machine under the supervision of the athletic trainer in the Department of Physical Education. This is Phase II of the rehabilitation program. The exercises are performed with both the injured and the unaffected leg. Evaluations are made at

* The Cybex II is the same machine that is used to measure the relative strengths of the quadriceps and hamstrings of each leg when a new cadet tells us that he has had a knee injury prior to entering West Point. This determines if the cadet requires a special conditioning program in order to bring the knees to comparable strength.

intervals of three weeks. At the end of twelve weeks the quadriceps and hamstrings have developed the additional strength that is necessary to expand their roles as secondary stabilizers for the injured knee.

During Phase II the athlete begins to develop and improve total athletic fitness by using strength, endurance, and flexibility exercises. As soon as the injured leg has redeveloped adequate range of motion in the knee, the athlete uses a stationary bicycle. Once the injured leg is 80 to 85 percent as strong as the good leg, a slow running program begins. This occurs four to six weeks into Phase II or about seven to nine weeks after surgery. Special attention is given to proper running mechanics, including guarding against pronation. The initial running distance is one-half to three-quarters of a mile unless there is pain or swelling. If that is the case, the running is reduced or postponed.

As the cadet's strength and confidence build, the running duration is increased one-half mile at a time. When the cadet is running steadily without pain, interval training is introduced to increase speed. The faster the cadet runs, the more stress is placed on the knee. However, if either pain or swelling occurs, a "step backward" is necessary. Remember that all rehabilitation steps are progressive, geared to what the leg can take.

Up to this point the running has been on a straight line. The cadet is concerned about what will happen when he makes sharp cuts and turns. The next sequence in the program is agility running, again with the cuts and turns graduated. The diagrams on page 238 are of a basketball court, illustrating the working of agility running progression. Note that the cuts and turns get tighter until in Chart 3 the tightest figure eight can be negotiated at top speed. Other agility drills are stair climbing—running up and walking down—reaction drills, and crossover steps. Rope skipping can also be used.

When major knee surgery is involved, the rehabilitation process takes from three to six months of hard, intensive work on the part of the cadet. The cadet is ready for competition when the following criteria are met:

  1. Bilateral strength of the injured leg is nearly equal (within 10 percent) to that of the good leg.

KNEE REHABILITATION
AGILITY RUNNING PROGRESSION

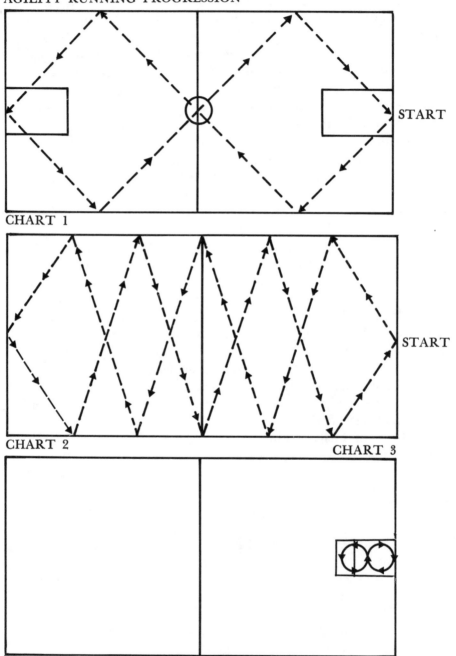

CHART 1

START

CHART 2   CHART 3

START

2. The anthropometric girth measurements of both thighs are nearly equal.

3. The integrity of the injured joint is established and asymptomatic when the cadet runs with speed and confidence, and when he cuts, turns, hops, and skips rope.

4. The orthopedic surgeon examines and clears the cadet to begin playing again.

This detailed example of comeback conditioning underlines the concept of total body integrity, as opposed to the disintegration of the whole because of an injury to a body part. Not all orthopedists are sympathetic to this concept. In fact, it is beyond the comprehension of some physicians.

One weekender recounted the experience of going to an orthopedist after a pain had been present in his foot for two weeks. The physician prescribed rest until the pain disappeared.

"I can't do that," the weekender said.

"What kind of work do you do?"

"I'm a writer."

The physician looked baffled.

"There should be no problem," he said. "Your work doesn't require you to be on your feet."

The writer explained that he had always been involved in physical activity and sports. What's more, he knew that he would feel "lousy" if he just sat around. The physician displayed neither sympathy nor understanding.

Under these circumstances anyone would do well to hunt down a sports physician. If that's impossible, discuss the problem with a doctor who also participates in weekend sports.

At the least, the injured weekender should continue with the program in the General Athletic Fitness and Special Athletic Fitness sections of this book, leaving out only those exercises that cause pain to the injured part. In the absence of professional advice, begin reconditioning at the lowest level when the pain and swelling are gone, using those exercises that relate to the injured part, and gradually bring the part back to full strength and flexibility.

The worst error is to quit exercising because you think you have to or because you are afraid of another injury. That is what the amateur philosopher would call "pennywise and pound foolish."

PART IV

The Physical Edge

*Specific Conditioning
for Specific Sports*

Chapter 16

SAF—Specific Athletic Fitness

The major factors in physical conditioning are the same for the professional and weekend athlete: Body composition, the ratio of body fat to lean body mass, determines functional efficiency. Virtually every athlete, including the superstars, must deal with the problem of overweight. The chief tool in coping with body composition is the intelligent application of nutritional information.

The second major factor is General Athletic Fitness, the foundation that prevents injuries and provides the endurance to outlast your opponent. See Part III, "The Winner's Circuit."

The third factor, discussed in this part of the book, is Specific Athletic Fitness, conditioning for specific body parts that improves game skills.

The conditioning, and it should always be quality conditioning, is the same for all athletes. The difference between the weekender and organized athletes is only a matter of time and intensity of effort. Organized athletes may know little about sports medicine but have the advantage of working many hours each day with a racquet, club, or ball which in itself develops a significant amount of specific conditioning, although not always enough to finish first and prevent injuries.

Weekend athletes by nature of their primary responsibilities spend most of their time in sedentary work. Grip-strength conditioning may be limited to the stress of holding a pen or shaking a hand, upper-torso strength to shrugging off some bad news, and lower-torso conditioning to standing and walking occasionally. There is nothing in the daily routine that contributes to the specific conditioning that improves skills in golf, tennis, or any other sport. Consequently the specific conditioning in this part of the book is critical to the weekender's performance. We guarantee that within your time limits the SAF program will give you a physical edge.

The Principle of Specificity Is Where the Action Is

No two physical activities require exactly the same mix of performance qualities. The graceful coordination sometimes demonstrated on a basketball court would look anything but graceful in a ballet studio—and vice versa. The mix in driving a golf ball differs from driving a softball or tennis ball. Anyone, including a star athlete, who goes directly from one sport to another wakes up the next morning with sore muscles or injuries. The athlete has ignored the principle of specificity. No matter that he was voted the most valuable player at the Super Bowl. He was out of condition for tennis.

Sports medicine has taught us that as much as possible Specific Athletic Fitness exercises should duplicate the exact conditions under which skills are ultimately going to be performed. For instance, the best way to learn tennis is to practice all the skills that are necessary to develop a complete game. However, if any quality is weak, such as the necessary grip strength to hold the racquet firmly, the skills cannot be properly practiced. So the weekender goes through life practicing mistakes.

The great athletes don't have this problem. Most of them, including the top-seeded players, travel with personal coaches in constant attendance. Under a coach's eye mistakes are corrected instantly. The pro is forced to include the proper mix of performance factors in play. Although this is not the most efficient way of developing strength and flexibility, it works. Of course, the weekend athlete has neither the luxury of personal coaching nor long hours to spend on the court. But the weekender has a shortcut to developing skills by taking advantage of the research in specific conditioning.

Now that sports medicine has identified the biological systems involved in different sports, we can recommend specific motor performance. Furthermore, we can identify the level of conditioning required in muscular strength and endurance, cardiorespiratory endurance, flexibility, speed, and agility. This is the technology, the practical application of sports medicine, that you will find in this part of the book.

We understand that the weekender's time is so limited that getting into high-intensity training would be an indulgence. With the time limitation in mind, we have identified the most significant weakness of the average weekend athlete sport by sport and prescribed programs that will correct these weaknesses.

For the purpose of organization more than anything else, the different sports have been grouped in the following three categories:

1. Individual Sports
   a. Vigorous conditioning sports
   b. Recreational sports
2. Dual Sports
   a. Dual/court sports
   b. Dual/combative sports
3. Team Sports

Before you turn to your favorite sport, there is one other important matter to be dealt with—the complexity of juggling GAF and SAF workouts with games.

In-Season Fitness Schedule for the Weekend Athlete

The General Athletic Fitness program is your power base, but it also ensures your health. This is one good argument for maintaining general fitness year around. In addition, when your sport comes into season, you won't have to sweat up a storm to shape up.

During the period when your sport is out of season, as few as three workouts a week on alternate days will maintain body tone. About six weeks before your game comes into season begin working on the Special Athletic Fitness program to improve skills demanded by the sport. Increase workouts to six days a week, alternating the GAF and SAF programs. So far, so good.

The breakdown in conditioning occurs when the playing season begins because there are now three physical elements to contend with—GAF, SAF, and games—and that's when both the professional and weekend athlete make the same error. During the playing season there is a tendency to concentrate on SAF conditioning to improve skills. If you then neglect GAF, your overall strength and endurance drop, concentration falters, and the competitive edge

On a Scale of 1 to 10 . . .

COMPONENT RATINGS FOR 33 SPORTS

	Muscular Strength		Muscular Endurance		Agility	Coordination	Reaction time	Flexibility		Cardio-Respiratory Endurance	Body Composition (Lean Weight vs. Fat Weight)
	Upper Body	*Lower Body*	*Upper Body*	*Lower Body*				*Upper Body*	*Lower Body*		
Individual Sports											
Archery	5	4	5	4	0	2	3	5	2	0	3
Bicycling	2	7	2	10	0	0	1	0	5	10	5
Bowling	4	3	4	4	4	5	2	5	5	1	4
Fishing	3	5	4	5	4	5	5	4	5	3	4
Golf	7	5	7	7	2	8	4	7	6	3	5
Horseback Riding	5	5	5	5	2	2	5	4	4	2	5
Ice Skating	2	6	2	8	5	5	2	5	7	7	5
Mountaineering	8	8	7	8	5	4	3	7	7	5	7
Roller Skating	2	6	2	8	5	5	2	5	7	7	5
Running/Jogging	2	6	2	10	4	4	1	2	6	10	8
Scuba Diving	5	5	8	7	3	3	1	5	5	8	4

VERY LOW 0 — LOW 1 — 2 — BELOW AVERAGE 3 — 4 — AVERAGE 5 — ABOVE AVERAGE 6 — 7 — HIGH 8 — 9 — VERY HIGH 10

	1	2	3	4	5	6	7	8	9	10	11
Skiing:											
Cross-Country	7	8	7	10	5	6	3	7	7	10	8
Downhill	6	6	5	8	7	7	5	7	8	6	5
Swimming	7	5	8	8	5	5	3	5	5	10	4
Water Skiing	7	6	8	8	5	5	5	5	6	6	5
Weight Lifting	10	10	8	8	5	4	5	7	7	5	6
Dual/Court Sports											
Badminton	4	5	5	5	5	6	5	6	6	5	5
Handball	5	5	6	7	7	7	5	6	8	8	7
Paddle Tennis	5	5	6	6	6	7	5	6	7	7	6
Platform Tennis	5	5	6	6	6	7	5	6	7	7	6
Racquetball/Paddle Ball	5	5	6	7	7	7	5	6	8	8	7
Squash	5	6	6	7	8	8	6	6	8	8	7
Tennis	5	7	7	8	6	8	5	6	7	8	7
Dual/Combative											
Fencing	5	5	5	5	5	5	6	5	5	4	6
Judo	9	9	9	6	6	5	6	8	8	6	4
Karate	9	9	9	6	5	5	5	7	8	6	5
Team Sports											
Baseball/Softball	7	6	7	5	6	8	5	7	6	3	6
Basketball	5	8	6	9	8	7	5	6	7	8	7
Soccer	5	8	2	9	8	8	6	5	8	9	7
Touch Football	5	7	6	5	5	5	4	7	6	5	5
Volleyball	6	8	5	8	9	8	6	8	9	4	7

dulls. To counter this falloff in performance, the following schedules are suggested:

In-Season Workout Schedule
For Moderate and Heavy Activity Sports

Sunday	Game	GAF	SAF
Monday	GAF	SAF	Game
Tuesday	SAF	Game	GAF
Wednesday	Game	GAF	Game
Thursday	GAF	Game	SAF
Friday	SAF	SAF	Game
Saturday	Game	Game	GAF

q

Note: The above schedule is designed for the weekender who plays three days a week, allowing two days for GAF and two for SAF. If you play fewer than three days, you may opt to use the open day to rest or to work on your weakest area—GAF, SAF, cardiorespiratory conditioning, or flexibility.

In-Season Workout Schedule
For Light Activity Sports

Sunday	Game	GAF	SAF
Monday	GAF	Game	Rest
Tuesday	Rest	Rest	Game
Wednesday	SAF	SAF	GAF
Thursday	Rest	Game	Rest
Friday	GAF	GAF	GAF
Saturday	Game	Rest	Game

r

Note: The above schedule requires two GAF and one SAF days as minimum conditioning. You may opt to use the rest days for either a game or cardiorespiratory conditioning, flexibility, or a full session of SAF.

Chapter 17

Individual Sports

Aquatic Sports
Archery
Backpacking and Climbing
Bicycling
Bowling
Fishing
Golf
Horseback Riding
Ice Skating
Roller Skating
Running/Jogging
Snow Skiing
Weight Lifting

Although primarily recreational, individual sports offer a variety of benefits. Most can be used to develop health, and most can be made competitive, against either other players or a personal set of standards. Scuba diving is the exception unless you consider speargun fishing competitive. Mountaineering may be recreational or intensely competitive, the individual against mountain.

The individual sports with their activity levels—light (L), moderate (M), or high (H)—are:

Aquatic Sports
   Scuba Diving (M)
   Skin Diving (M)
   Swimming (H)
   Water Skiing (H)
Archery (L)
Bicycling (M)

Bowling (L)
Fishing (L)
Golf (L)
Horseback Riding (L)
Ice Skating (M)
Mountaineering (H)
Roller Skating (M)
Running/Jogging (H)
Skiing:
   Cross-Country (H)
   Downhill (M)
Weight Lifting (H)

Aquatic Sports: scuba diving, skin diving, swimming, water skiing

Swimming is unique in modern culture. It is the world's most popular sport and the only sport that provides the body with total conditioning. It is both a recreational and survival art. Curiously swimming as we know it today, a highly developed and competitive sport, is a latecomer in the context of sports history.

Swimming is an acquired skill, and ancient cave drawings tell us that prehistoric man learned to swim. Greek and Roman warriors used swimming as a fitness conditioner. Ancient Assyrian bas-reliefs show soldiers swimming streams. At West Point today a cadet must qualify in survival swimming as a prerequisite to graduating. The cadet's proficiency must include the ability to swim 24 yards with a 10-pound brick in battle dress carrying a rifle and backpack. None of this may sound surprising, but for several hundred years swimming was forbidden throughout the Western world.

During the Middle Ages outdoor bathing was thought to be a major cause of the spread of disease. It was virtually outlawed until the 1880's, when Great Britain brought back organized swimming competition. Since then swimming has come to be recognized as a major event in international competition, second only to track.

Many weekend athletes are drawn to swimming for the relaxation and buoyancy that occur only in water and outer space. The serious swimmer, as distinguished from the paddlers, gains exceptional conditioning benefits. Swimming brings into play more muscles than any other exercise. In addition, it is an excellent cardiorespiratory conditioner, although most swimmers don't know how to apply CR guidelines.

Being a good swimmer is not a requirement in learning to water ski or dive, but good swimming skills are critical in emergency situations. Although specific conditioning will be recommended for skiing and diving, the bottom line in all aquatic sports is swimming. Therefore, swimming is emphasized as the basic activity.

BODY PARTS

Swimming requires general body conditioning. The most important body parts are the muscles of the shoulders, chest, and upper back (shoulder girdle); the upper arms, front and back; and the hip flexors. In addition, the cardiorespiratory system is highly important.

CONDITIONING

The conditioning is required for all aquatic sports. Only diving is not rated as a heavy activity at a recreational level. However, good physical fitness is absolutely essential for divers who may have to cope with life-threatening situations. During such emergencies you may not be able to rely on support equipment. Swimming skills and physical fitness become your only means of survival.

1. General Athletic Fitness. The GAF conditioning program can be used to maintain conditioning during the off-season, to prepare for a warm-water vacation during the winter, or to supplement your conditioning during the aquatic season.

Only a few years ago people thought activities such as weight training, calisthenics, and running were counterproductive in preparing a person to swim. Sports research has taught us better. Today our best swimmers are using calisthenics and weight training to improve their performance and go for the gold. Although the best way to develop cardiorespiratory fitness for swimming is by swimming, it is not the only way—and not the preferable way when the pond is frozen over.

Weekenders who have year-round access to a pool may use swimming as a cardiorespiratory conditioner if they follow a few simple rules.

To develop cardiorespiratory fitness, you must swim vigorously enough to bring your pulse rate to at least 60 percent and preferably 70 percent of your MHR (maximum heart rate). Your MHR is estimated by subtracting your age from 220. If you are age 40, your MHR would be 180 (220—40 = 180). Then 70 percent of 180, your MHR, gives you 126, which is your conditioning rate.

There are several good body spots to take your pulse. The two most commonly used are the wrist and neck. (See illustration on page 253.) Look for your arterial pulse on the thumb side of your wrist or on either side of your Adam's apple.

After you get swimming vigorously, stop briefly, and immediately take your pulse for a count of 6 seconds. Add a zero to the count, and this will give you a workable reading of your heart rate. You must then maintain your pulse rating at better than 60 or 70 percent of MHR for a period of 12 minutes or longer if it is to count as a cardiorespiratory conditioner. You may discover that you have to be a fairly strong swimmer to maintain your pulse rate at a conditioning level. This is one reason why you should work at the GAF Level III before the swimming season gets under way or before you undertake other aquatic sports.

For strong swimmers and water skiers, the workout should be at GAF Level III. Do not neglect the stretching exercises in the warm-up and cool-down phases. Flexibility is a worthwhile precaution for the water skier who wants to avoid the stiff neck and sore shoulder that result from a high-speed fall.

Diving enthusiasts, either skin or scuba, must realize that the activity itself contributes very little to their conditioning level. When underwater, movements must be slow and efficient in order to conserve air supply. Therefore, you must develop conditioning in order to dive safely and enjoyably. For the average weekend diver, GAF Level II is adequate. However, if you are going to dive in remote areas where chances of emergencies are high, conditioning at GAF Level III is recommended.

2. Specific Athletic Fitness.

a. During the swimming season continue with GAF Level III workouts at least twice each week, immediately before swimming, if convenient. In addition, plan a daily turn with the GAF flexibility exercises 1, 2, or 3; or 4, 5, 7, 8, 9, and 10. These stretch exercises should also be performed before and after each swim session.

b. During the water skiing season continue the GAF Level III

TWO MOST COMMON PULSE SITES

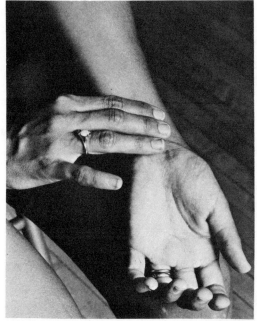

RADIAL ARTERY

CAROTID ARTERY

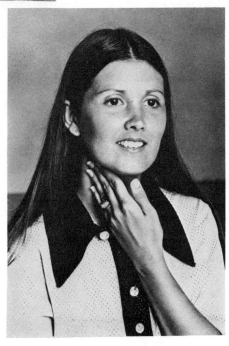

program at least three times per week on alternate days. At least once a week plan a swimming workout similar to a competitive event. Following is an example of such a workout that covers a total distance of 1,500 yards.

1,500-Yard Swimming Workout
1. Warm-up swim—200 yards.
2. Swim 4 x 100 yards on departure time of 2½ minutes.
3. Swim 200 yards—continuous swim.
4. Kick* 200 yards—then kick 2 x 50.
5. Pull † only 200 yards; then pull only 2 x 50.
6. Swim 6 x 50 on departure time of 1½ minutes.
Total distance = 1,500 yards.
Time estimate = approximately 1 hour.

Supplementary exercises prior to skiing should include GAF flexibility exercises 1, 2, or 3; or 4, 6, and 10 plus the other warm-up and cool-down exercises included in the GAF Level III program. Finally, you should also strengthen your grip with the Towel Twist exercise (see page 355).

c. During the skin and scuba diving season, continue the GAF Level II program at least three times per week, including the Extra Edge running program as a minimum supplement to the CR conditioning developed in the circuit training technique. Of course, you should also get in some vigorous swimming when you have the time and facilities. Prior to diving, be certain to do your stretching exercises; these would include 1, 2 or 3; or 4, 5, 6, and 7.

HEALTH AND FITNESS ANALYSIS

1. The three aquatic activities will result in the average 117- or 150-pound person's burning calories as follows:

	Calories per Hour	
	117-pound Person	*150-pound Person*
Swimming	475 calories	570 calories
Scuba/skin		
Diving	450 calories	540 calories
Water skiing	365 calories	475 calories

* Use only legs for propulsion.
† Use only arms for propulsion.

2. Swimming and water skiing are classified as heavy-activity sports. Scuba/skin diving at the recreational level rates as a moderate-activity sport.

a. Swimming is recommended for anyone of any age who has learned swimming skills. Swimming can be learned at any age with certain reservations. Those with a phobic fear of swimming will require expert instruction. Older people with hydrophobia may suffer excessive psychological stress and should pick up the phone and consult their physicians before taking the plunge.

b. Scuba and skin diving are activities that should be approached warily by people over 45 who have never dived at a younger age and who are out of practice and condition.

c. Water skiing is also an activity for the relatively young who have maintained their conditioning and kept up the activity. For the normal person, the age of 45 should be the limit.

3. Recreational and skin/scuba diving does not require the high levels of muscular strength and endurance that are necessary for competitive swimming. Swimming by itself will not develop strength, but it will increase muscular endurance of the arms, shoulders, and legs. The strength will be developed in the GAF program.

For water skiing, grip strength and arm and shoulder strength and endurance are required at a higher level than for diving and swimming. In addition, the quadriceps, groin muscles, and hamstrings receive more stress.

4. Swimming is an excellent cardiorespiratory activity, but diving and water skiing are not. However, conditioning is necessary if you are going to excel at these activities.

Archery The prehistoric invention of the bow is considered one of society's most important cultural advances, equivalent to the development of speech and the making of fire. The bow is an ingenious mechanical device in which energy can be gradually accumulated, stored temporarily, and then instantly released to project a missile with greater accuracy than any other device except the firearm.

The bow and arrow were the major instrument of the hunter and warrior until the invention of the gun in the sixteenth century. Since then archery has been a favorite sport of kings and Robin

Hoods, and today it enjoys widespread popularity with both men and women, as a competitive and recreational sport. Archery is challenging. It requires the coordination of muscles and mind, a cool demeanor, and a sharp eye.

Modern competitive bows are classified according to the draw weight, the weight of pull when the bow is at full draw. In competition, the draw weight is between 35 and 45 pounds for men, 24 to 28 pounds for women. Men shoot at distances of 30, 50, 70, and 90 meters; women, at 30, 50, 60, and 70 meters. Lighter bows, for children and beginners, draw at 15 to 25 pounds. Lighter bows are always recommended for beginners until skills and strength are developed.

BODY PARTS

Much of the work in drawing the bow is performed in the arm and shoulder-girdle area. This includes the muscles of the upper back, such as the trapezius and rhomboids, which help stabilize and pull the scapulae together. Also important are the muscles of the shoulders and upper arms, especially the deltoids.

Archery requires the ability to apply strength in drawing the bow while remaining relaxed in order to aim the arrow skillfully into the white core of the target. Concentration is of the utmost importance as is smooth well-coordinated movement.

CONDITIONING

Special attention should be given to the flexibility exercises of the back and shoulders (8, 9, 10) while continuing and maintaining overall conditioning at GAF Level I.

HEALTH AND FITNESS ANALYSIS

Archery is a light-activity sport that all age-groups can enjoy.

A 117-pound person will burn up about 240 calories per hour of participation; a 150-pound person, about 310 calories.

Archery injuries are minor. If finger tabs or finger gloves are not used, blisters normally occur on the fingers that draw the bowstring. Similarly, the forearm may be bruised near the wrist if armguards are not worn or if the wrist and forearm of the archer are not strong enough to maintain a firm wrist when the bow is drawn.

The cardiorespiratory fitness required for archery is the same as required for basic fitness. The level developed in following the program in GAF Level I is adequate.

Backpacking and Climbing Backpacking ran range from an easy hike through the forest to mountain climbing, when provisions for a week or longer must be carried on your back. Climbing may also range from an easy walk up gentle slopes without a backpack to belayed climbing on difficult rock faces. The more difficult the climbing, the more dangerous and the more unforgiving the mistakes. At this time your level of conditioning is most important. When your opponent is the mountain, the difference between winning and losing is somewhat dramatic.

BODY PARTS

Backpacking and climbing require total body conditioning. The level depends on the size of the mountain. Flexibility of the arms, shoulders, backs, thighs, lower legs, and ankles is important. Strength and muscular endurance of the arms and shoulder girdle, upper and lower back, abdomen, thighs, calves, shins, ankles, and grip strength are vital. Cardiorespiratory conditioning is extremely important if you are to maintain your stamina.

Most common injuries, including Achilles tendonitis, shin splints, sciatica, and arch or heel pain, can be prevented by proper conditioning. Such other common injuries as blisters and calluses are usually caused by improper shoe fit. Falls may be the result of poor technique, equipment, judgment, or conditioning. However, poor conditioning often begets a lack of self-confidence, and those who lack confidence will normally not put themselves in a dangerous position.

The goal in the development of upper-body strength should be the capacity to lift and hold your body weight using only your hands and arms. This applies to both men and women. This is a prerequisite for anyone who wants to climb. For those who limit their backpacking to nature trails, a lower level of upper-body strength is adequate.

CONDITIONING

1. General Athletic Fitness conditioning for the weekend hiker/

climber should be at GAF Level III. For the serious climber, cardio-respiratory conditioning is recommended in the Extra Edge program. You may choose to do this by alternating the Circuit Training one day and the Extra Edge running program the next. On running days include the Specific Athletic Fitness program noted below. Two days of circuit and two days of running/SAF per week are adequate. However, three days of each per week are preferable if you have the time. If the climb is difficult, make the time!

2. The SAF program when used in conjunction with GAF Level III will provide the conditioning to make mountain climbing possible, enjoyable and safe.

Warm Up/Flexibility (Flexibility exercises 1, 3, 6, and 7 on pages 98, 102, 108, 110.)

Bent-Knee Sit-ups (see page 160).

PULL-UPS

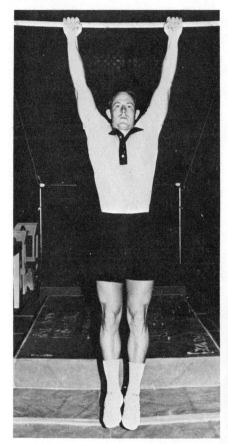

STARTING
POSITION

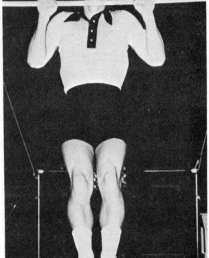

COUNT 1

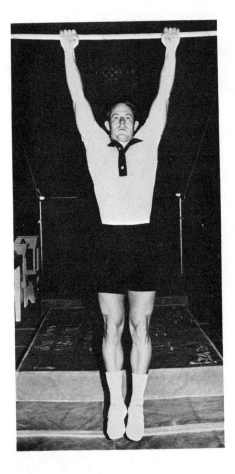

COUNT 2

Pull-Ups

Starting Position: Hang from a 1½-inch-diameter horizontal bar
   that is high enough to lift your feet off the ground, palms face
   forward, hands about shoulder width apart.

Action: Count 1: Pull up your body until your chin is above the
   bar.

   Count 2: Lower your body until your arms are fully extended and you have returned to the starting position.

Cadence: Moderate.

Progression: Do as many pull-ups as possible. If you do fewer than
   7, continue by doing Negative Pull-ups.

NEGATIVE PULL-UPS

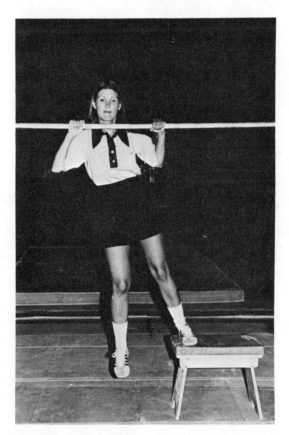

GETTING INTO THE STARTING POSITION

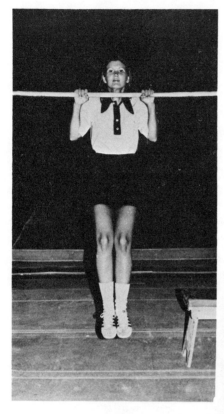

STARTING POSITON

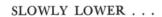

SLOWLY LOWER . . .

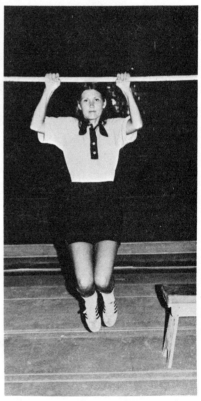

Negative Pull—ups

Starting Position: Use a chair or stool to raise yourself to the position where you will begin with your chin above the bar and your arms and hands prepared to support you. Step off the stool.

Action: Count 1: As slowly as you can, gradually lower your body until your arms are fully extended and you are hanging freely from the bar.

Count 2: Use the stool/chair again to return to the starting position with your chin over the bar.

Cadence: Very slow. Take a minimum of 4 seconds to lower your body, longer, if possible.

Progression: Continue doing Negative Pull-ups until your arms will no longer support your weight. (*Note*: West Point has experimented with a number of methods to develop pull-up ability. The negative pull-up is the most successful method. It works for both men and women.)

TOE LIFT

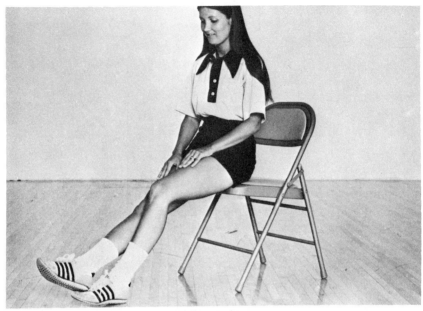

STARTING POSITION (LEFT FOOT)

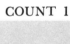

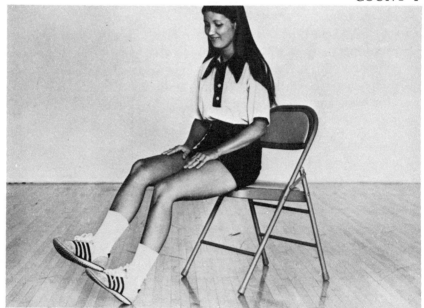

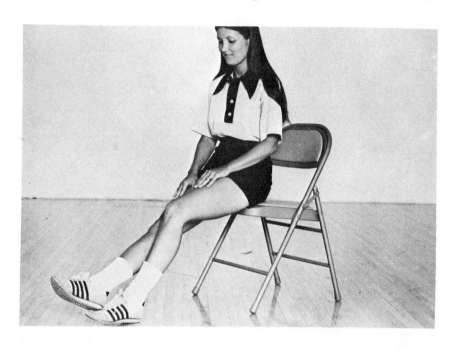

STARTING POSITION (RIGHT FOOT)

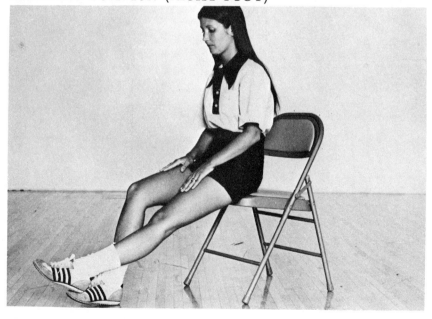

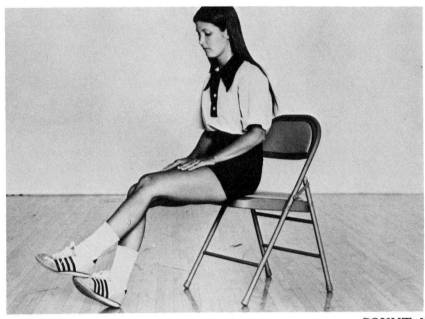

COUNT 1

COUNT 2

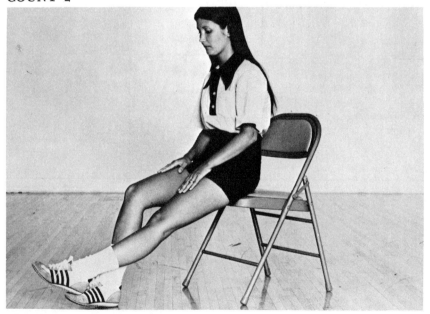

Toe Lift

Starting Position: Sit on a chair with the edge about 6 to 8 inches from the back of your knees. Half extend your legs with the heel of your left foot resting on the floor, your foot extended in a toe point. Place the heel of the right foot on the toes of the left foot.

Action: Count 1: While pressing your toes with the right heel, gradually flex your left foot as far as possible, and hold for 3 seconds.

Count 2: Release the pressure of the right heel, and return to the starting position.

Cadence: Very slow.

Progression: Start with 5 repetitions on both feet, and gradually increase to 10.

Ball Squeeze (see page 352).

Towel Twist (see page 355).

Note: Do all the above SAF exercises on the alternate days when you work out with the Extra Edge program described in GAF Level III.

3. Preactivity Warm-ups: Do flexibility exercises 1, 3, 6, and 7 shown on pages 98, 102, 108, 110. These exercises should be repeated after the climb.

HEALTH AND FITNESS ANALYSIS

1. When backpacking and carrying a 40-pound pack at 3 miles per hour, a 117-pound person will burn about 320 calories per hour; a 150-pound person, about 415 calories.

When mountain climbing, a 117-pound person will burn about 470 calories per hour; a 150-pound person about 605 calories.

2. Backpacking and mountain climbing are classified as heavy-activity sports.

3. This activity should be limited to the 12- to 60-year age-group. The exception is the person over 60 who has been climbing and backpacking routinely for many years. Backpacking is virtually impossible for youngsters and oldsters when you intend to go on a trail for five or six days. An individual pack cannot weigh less than 35

or 40 pounds. For older persons with back problems and in poor condition, a full pack is too much. Youngsters, despite their enthusiasm, will find backpacking difficult. In an experience with a group of Girl Scouts on the Long Trail in Vermont, the younger girls, including an 80-pound daughter, discovered that carrying a 30-pound backpack diminished the enjoyment of the trip. The rule for youngsters and oldsters: A hike in the woods, yes! A backpacking or climbing trip, no!

4. This activity demands good overall body muscular strength and endurance. Preparation for the season is an absolute must.

5. Cardiorespiratory fitness is also critical for long uphill climbs.

Bicycling   Bicycling began as cycling with man balanced above a single wheel and steering with his feet. As cycling evolved into a practical two-wheel machine capable of carrying both body and goods, the bicycle competed only with the horse. Self-propulsion lost its appeal for a time after the automobile appeared, but in the 1960's and 1970's the bicycle regained its mass popularity. In 1972 about 8.7 million bicycles were sold in the United States— the first time since the invention of the automobile that bicycle sales were greater than auto sales.

Bicycling can be competitive or a means of cardiorespiratory conditioning, but for most people it is recreational, popular with both sexes and all age-groups. In fact, some retirement communities provide adult-size tricycles for the health and enjoyment of senior citizens.

BODY PARTS

For the weekender, bicycling is an excellent aerobic activity, very effective in cardiorespiratory conditioning along with running and swimming.

Other body parts that get a heavy workout in bicycling include the muscles of the upper and lower legs: the quadriceps (front of the thighs), the calf muscles, and the Achilles tendons.

The shoulder and neck muscles contribute very little dynamic work. That is work that requires moving the body. However, the shoulders and neck perform considerable static work in supporting the weight of the head and the upper body.

Competitive bicycling is a heavy-activity sport that requires GAF conditioning at Level III. For weekenders not involved in competition, GAF Level II is appropriate.

SAF exercises take into consideration the need to maintain adequate flexibility during cycling. For the thighs, use the Step-ups (page 166) as shown in GAF Level III. For the calf muscles, use the Elevated Toe Raisers (page 152) in GAF Level II. Stretching exercises should include 1, 2, 5, 7, 8, and 9. Exercises 1, 2, and 5 compensate for the cycling tendency to shorten leg muscles. Exercise 7 helps maintain the flexibility of the feet and ankles. Exercises 8 and 9 maintain flexibility of the upper back, neck, shoulders, and chest muscles. All these exercises, which take only a few minutes, should be performed before and after bicycling, to warm up and cool down.

Beginning cyclists experience neck pain or tired neck muscles because the neck muscles get little or no conditioning. Two exercises that can overcome this pain are:

WRESTLER'S BRIDGING

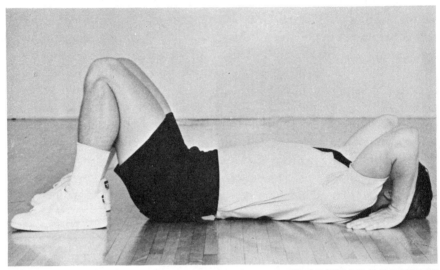

STARTING POSITION

COUNT 1

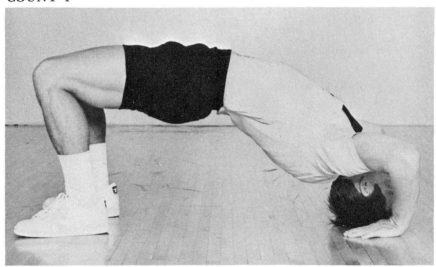

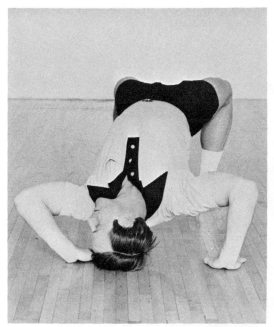

COUNT 2

COUNT 3

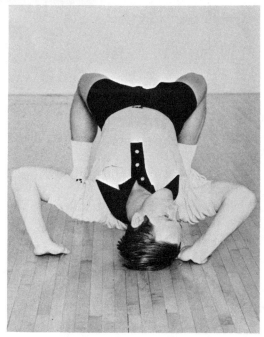

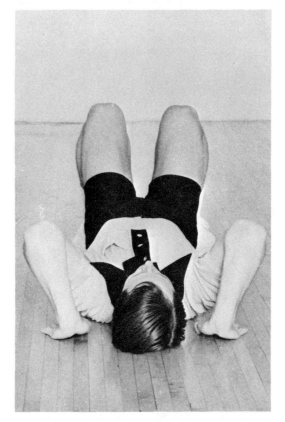

COUNT 4

1. *Wrestler's Bridging*

Starting Position: Lie on back with feet touching the buttocks, hands palms down on floor next to head with fingers pointing toward the body.

Action: Count 1: Pushing with hands and feet, raise the body until body weight is on the head and feet.

Count 2: Roll to the left.

Count 3: Roll to the right.

Count 4: Return to starting position.

Cadence: Slow.

Progression: Start with 5 repetitions, and gradually increase to 10 repetitions.

NECK EXTENSION

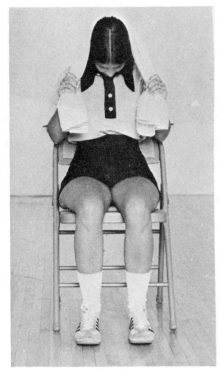

STARTING
POSITION

ACTION

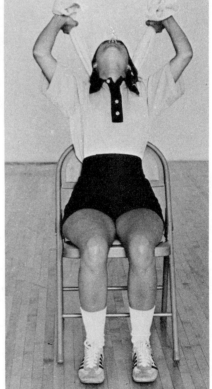

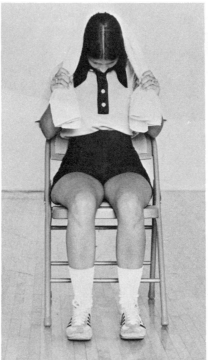

RETURN TO THE
STARTING
POSITION

2. Neck Extension

Starting Position: Sit in a hard chair with neck muscles relaxed
and chin on chest. Place a towel behind the head, and hold
the ends of the towel in your hands.

Action: Raise your chin off chest while applying pressure with
towel. Move your head up and back against the constant
pressure. (Pressure should be enough that neck muscles can
overcome the force.) Continue moving the head up and back
as far as it will go. At that point relax, and return to the
starting position. Repeat.

Cadence: Slow.

Progression: Start with 5 repetitions, and gradually increase to
12 repetitions.

HEALTH AND FITNESS ANALYSIS

1. Recreational bicycling by most weekend athletes is classified as a moderate activity; competitive racing, a heavy activity.

2. The recreational cyclist weighing 117 pounds will burn 234 calories per hour; the 150-pound cyclist, 306 calories.

The competitive cyclist weighing 117 pounds will burn 498 calories per hour; the 150-pound cyclist, 648 calories.

3. All age-groups can participate in recreational cycling. Competitive cycling is a sport for the younger set, normally under 30 years of age.

4. Although bicycling is an outstanding cardiorespiratory activity, muscular conditioning is limited to the thighs and hips. Note that stationary cycling is just as effective in CR conditioning as a road bicycle.

5. The bicycle seat should be raised in order that the leg is fully extended while pedaling. If the leg is not fully extended, the quadriceps muscles never get a chance to relax and thus become sore. In the fully extended position, you should be pressing against the pedals with the balls of your feet, not the instep.

There is little chance of injury in cycling, except for accidents. When riding in heavy traffic, wear padded headgear.

Bowling As far back as the Stone Age *Homo erectus* rolled rocks at pointed stones. Ancient Polynesians rolled egg-shaped balls in an "alley" 60 feet long, the same distance used in tenpin bowling today. About 7,000 years ago the Egyptians were playing at tenpins.

So many people find bowling irresistible that in the thirteenth century Edward III introduced into England a law forbidding bowling because it interfered with the practice of archery, which was then critical to national defense. However, Henry VIII, a world-class archer, installed bowling alleys at Whitehall to satisfy his passion for the pins. And it is reported that Sir Francis Drake refused to break up a bowling game despite being notified of the approach of the Spanish Armada.

No one can question the fascination of bowling. It is challenging and competitive but is not a sport that promotes fitness. The physical exertion required in a foursome match is less than the energy put into a slow stroll around the block. On the other hand, the bowler is well served by conditioning in order to avoid some of the common aches and pains that directly result from bowling.

BODY PARTS

In bowling the same movements are repeated over and over again. This makes the game easy to learn. The problem is in the one-sided action. The heavy work in one arm throws the other side of the body out of balance. This twists the lower back and leads to low-back pain. The twisting, bending movement also puts undue stress on the knees.

Another problem is bowler's hip, caused by the repeated hip extension along with the twisting motion of the lower back. This action may cause inflammation of the iliopsoas tendon where it attaches to the femur. Although this is not a serious injury, it can result in a very annoying deep hip pain when one walks, runs, or climbs stairs.

CONDITIONING

The aches and pains noted above are the bane of the sedentary adult. Bowling is such a light activity that GAF conditioning at Level I will adequately prepare you for bowling and protect you from morning-after discomfort. However, you should continue the GAF conditioning throughout the bowling season because the sport itself will not keep you in shape.

Work out a minimum of two times per week, preferably at least three times on alternate days, but not more than four. Schedule your conditioning sessions on days when you are not bowling. When running in place, concentrate on lifting your knees high. This will help strengthen the iliopsoas and thereby counter-act the continual hip extension that causes bowler's hip.

Note: Bowler's thumb cannot be prevented by conditioning. This problem usually is caused by a ball that is too heavy for the bowler or grip holes that are too small, thus exerting too much friction on the thumb. The solution is to get a lighter ball and better fit. A tip to the beginner: Start with a lighter ball—men, 14 pounds; women, 10 pounds.

HEALTH AND FITNESS ANALYSIS

1. Bowling is a light-activity sport.

2. A 150-pound bowler in a foursome will burn 210 calories per hour; a 117-pound bowler, 162 calories.

3. As with all light-activity sports, all age-groups and sexes can participate in bowling.

4. The muscular strength and endurance required of the bowler are minimal, no more than the level of a normal, healthy person who can claim adequate basic fitness.

5. There is no cardiorespiratory conditioning benefit in bowling.

Fishing The world's most popular and beloved sport is fishing. A light activity, it has little value as a conditioner, but conditioning contributes to the comfort and skills of the fisherman.

The fly fisherman, just as the golfer, requires grip, arm, and shoulder strength, and if a favorite stream requires a hard hike, there's a real need for lower-torso fitness. Deep-sea fishing is considerably more strenuous, demanding a strong trunk and back and strong arms, shoulders, and hands. On the other hand, the pond fisherman who sits on the bank or a drifting boat barely needs enough strength to suppress a yawn or swat away a fly.

BODY PARTS

The critical body parts, except for the sitting fisherman, include the legs for hiking and standing, the trunk to stabilize the pelvic girdle when walking and standing for long periods of time, and the arm, shoulder, and handgrip to manipulate fishing tackle. Handgrip is likely to be the most important on a long day whether you are fishing in fresh or salt water. Injury and risk are virtually nonexistent if you fish only with experienced people and if you stay out of the way of the hooks when they are being cast and are not careless when removing the hooks from your catch.

CONDITIONING

Adequate physical fitness for fishing can be maintained by exercising at GAF Level I, Progression Step 1 and working up to Progression Step 3. For the average fisherman, no further conditioning is necessary. However, for the deep-sea fisherman or the freshwater fisherman who goes after the big ones, such as a largemouth bass, some specific work on the grip strength is helpful.

In addition to the GAF Level I program, specific conditioning may include grip strength conditioning. See page 351.

See page 351.

HEALTH AND FITNESS ANALYSIS

1. Except for hiking and lugging a boat, motor, and other equipment, fishing classifies as a light-activity sport.

2. A fisherman weighing 117 pounds will burn about 192 calories per hour on the average; a 150-pound person, about 240 calories.

3. All age-groups and sexes can enjoy fishing, although a person with high blood pressure should have the approval of a cardiologist before engaging in deep-sea fishing.

4. Fishing does not require unusual muscular strength and endurance except the patience to endure a day when the fish don't bite.

5. In fishing itself there is no cardiorespiratory conditioning benefit.

Golf No one knows when golf originated in Scotland, but three times during the fourteenth century the Scottish Parliament decreed that golf "be utterly cryed downe, and not to be used" because of the game's interference with the public's normal duties. Today, five centuries later, tens of thousands of adults are still being sucked out of their homes by an obsessive need to test their skills on a ball that's barely the size of a plum. The golfer accepts his fate. The golf widow has no recourse.

To the casual observer the golf course appears to be an environment of absolute tranquillity. Sunlight glosses manicured greenery, and the players appear to be enjoying a stroll that's interrupted occasionally by hitting the little ball. It's all very deceptive and belies the intensity that crushes the heart of a golfer. The compulsion to putt the tiny moonlike object into a hole at the trifling distance of 3 feet is more overwhelming at that instant than the challenge of putting the first man on the moon.

The intensity of the golfer is totally contradicted by the physical demands of the game. An equivalent amount of physical conditioning can be found in sunbathing. This is especially true today, when many courses require golf carts to speed up playing, eliminating walking and carrying a bag.

Golf is a light activity. Even the energy required to swing a club from 70 to 100 or more times during a round is negligible when you consider that more than one-third of the strokes occur on the green, requiring the light touch of a putter. Still, the intensity and concentration depend on fitness, and the physical movements depend on conditioning.

BODY PARTS

The golfer's most important body parts are the arms and shoulders, the hands, and the trunk. Include the legs if the golfer walks and carries the clubs.

Some of the golfer's more common aches and pains include the golfer's knee and low-back pain. These problems are normally the result of poor conditioning or failure to warm up properly before play.

CONDITIONING

GAF conditioning at Level I will help prevent the aches and pains noted above and at the same time add 20 or 30 yards to your drive. Improving your grip strength will drive the ball farther (see the Ball Squeeze and Towel Twisting exercises on pages 352 and 355).

Flexibility is very important to the golfer. There are several exercises that take less than five minutes that should be done daily.

GOLFER'S TRUNK TWISTER

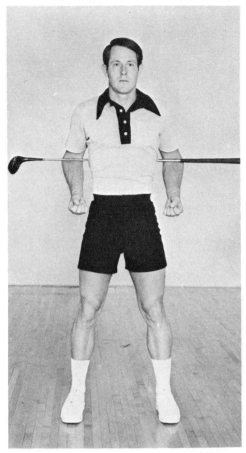

STARTING POSITION

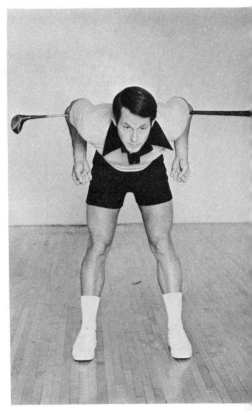

COUNT 1

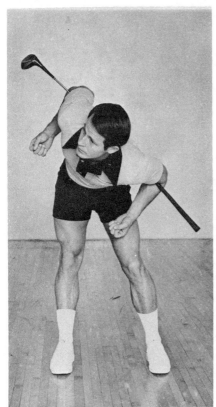

COUNT 2

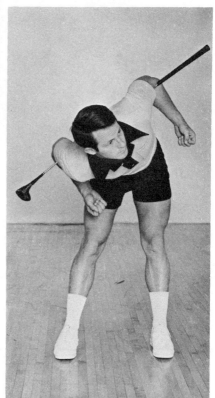

COUNT 3

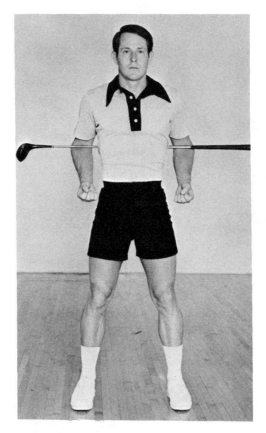

COUNT 4

Golfer's Trunk Twister

Starting Position: Stand with feet about shoulder width apart. Hold a golf club in place across your back by supporting it in the crooks of your elbows.

Action: Count 1: Bend forward at the waist until the back is parallel with the ground. (*Note*: this exercise can also be performed without bending at the waist.)

Count 2: Twist the trunk to the right.

Count 3: Twist the trunk to the left.

Count 4: Return to the starting position.

Cadence: Moderate to slow.

Progression: Begin with 6 repetitions, and gradually increase to 12.

The other recommended flexibility exercises for the golfer are the four prescribed in the GAF Level I program plus the Shoulders Stretch (see page 115, Exercise 10). A golf club may be used instead of a towel.

Pregame conditioning is just as important to the golfer as it is for athletes who play moderate- and heavy-activity sports. A good warm-up ritual for the golfer should include:

1. At home or in the locker room, work through the four warm-up/flexibility exercises in GAF Level I.

2. On the golf course, before hitting any balls, use the Shoulder Stretch with Golf Club or Towel and the Golfer's Trunk Twister.

3. Take some practice swings with your short irons (7, 8, or 9) before beginning to swing your woods. Ideally, go to the practice tee, and hit some practice balls, using first the short irons and then the woods.

HEALTH AND FITNESS ANALYSIS

1. Playing in a foursome, a 117-pound person will burn 192 calories per hour; a 150-pound person, 246 calories.

2. Golf is a light-activity sport.

3. All age-groups and both sexes can play golf.

4. Golf does not require exceptional strength or endurance, but a golfer must be in good physical condition to play up to his capability.

5. Cardiorespiratory fitness above that required by any healthy person is not required for golf. However, as with any competitive sport, the muscles can work effectively only if the cardiorespiratory system delivers oxygen to the essential muscle groups.

Horseback Riding Horseback riding is a good muscle conditioner for the horse, and riding at a canter or gallop is an excellent aerobic activity for the horse. However, for most weekenders, riding is a light activity that in itself contributes little to fitness. Instead, the weekender should use conditioning to be prepared for the specific demands made by the horse.

BODY PARTS

The rider's most important muscle groups are the adductor muscles on the inside of the thighs. These muscles perform the work of squeezing the legs together, a very important action when riding. Other muscle groups called into action are those of the trunk, including the abdomen, the calf muscles, and the Achilles tendons.

Common injuries in riding other than from a fall, include ruptured adductor muscles, or groin pull, and the sequel to ruptured adductors, calcification within the inflamed muscle tissue.

CONDITIONING

1. General Athletic Fitness. General conditioning should be at least at GAF Level I. Special attention should be given to the Achilles tendon stretch (page 98). Achilles tendons are in a stretched position in the stirrups with the toes higher than the heels.

2. Specific Athletic Fitness. The weekend rider who faithfully follows the GAF Level I program does not need to work at any higher level to be in condition for riding. However, since the leg adductor muscles are used in a contracted state when riding, it is important that they be stretched routinely. Two flexibility exercises are recommended to stretch the groin muscles (adductors longus, magnus, brevis, and minimus and the gracilis and pectineus).

STANDING GROIN STRETCH

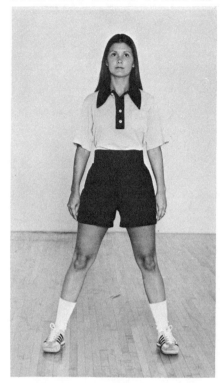

STARTING
POSITION

COUNT 1

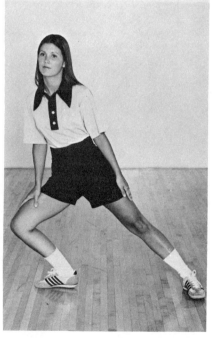

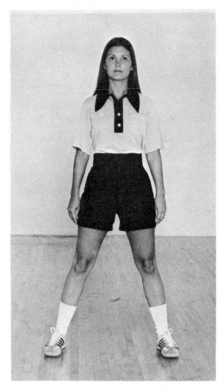

COUNT 2

COUNT 3

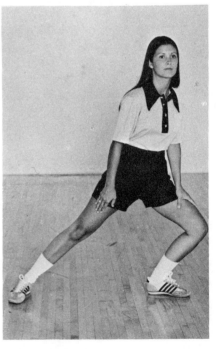

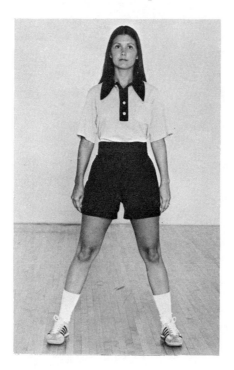

COUNT 4

Standing Groin Stretch

Starting Position: Stand with feet spread slightly wider than shoulder width with hands on hips, toes pointing straight ahead.

Action: Count 1: Turn the right toe out at a 45-degree angle, and bend the right knee as you lean your trunk to the right until you feel the stretch in the groin of the left leg. Hold the stretch for 10 to 15 seconds.

Count 2: Return to the starting position with the right toe pointing straight ahead.

Count 3: Turn the left toe out, and repeat Count 1 on the left side.

Count 4: Return to the starting position.

Cadence: Slow.

Progression: Begin with 5 repetitions, and gradually increase to 10. Also increase the amount of stretch gradually by spreading the legs farther apart, and hold the stretch for up to 30 seconds.

GROIN PRESS

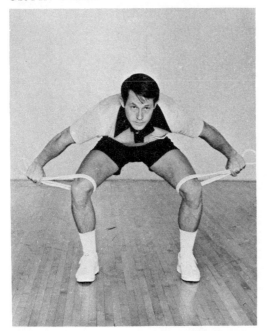

STARTING POSITION

ACTION

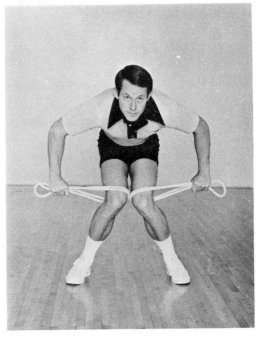

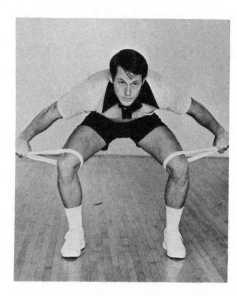

RETURN TO
STARTING
POSITION

Groin Press

Starting Position: Lean against a wall, refrigerator, or file cabinet
with feet spread about 24 inches, toes pointing directly to the
front and elevated about 2 inches above the heels. (A 2-inch
board, book, or brick can be used.) The knees should be
slightly bent, and the trunk slightly flexed. Wrap a belt or
towel around each knee. Hold the ends of the towels firmly to
the outside of the knees.

Action: Using the belts/towels to resist the action, gradually try to
press the knees and thighs together. Work through the full
range of motion until the thighs or knees touch. (*Note*: This
exercise can be somewhat duplicated by using a large ball, the
size of a basketball or beach ball. Holding the ball between the
knees, press the legs into the ball for 5 to 10 seconds, and release. Be advised that this version of the exercise is completely
isometric and can cause your blood pressure to rise significantly.)

Cadence: Very slow.

Progression: Begin with 5 repetitions, and gradually build up to 10.

Groin Stretch (see Exercise 6, page 108)

Another important SAF exercise for the weekend rider is the Bent-Knee Curl or the Bent-Knee Sit-up. These exercises can be found in the GAF section at GAF Level II and III, respectively. You may begin with the Bent-Knee Curl and then substitute the Sit-up when you feel ready.

3. Preactivity Warm-ups: As a minimum, the weekend rider should warm up by doing the Achilles Stretch (page 98) and the Groin Stretch (page 108) or the Standing Groin Stretch (page 285).

HEALTH AND FITNESS ANALYSIS

1. A 117-pound person will burn about 180 calories per hour, and a 150-pound person, 240 calories during a weekend ride. The horse will do considerably better.

2. Riding for the typical weekend rider is a light-activity sport. For the rider involved in a hunt or competitive jumping, riding is a moderate activity because the large muscle groups of the legs and trunk are called into play.

3. Riding is open to the healthy person of any age, keeping in mind that most injuries occur while mounting and dismounting. Those who have lost suppleness and agility should be helped getting on and off a horse. It is not recommended that people who have lost confidence in their agility and balance should contemplate learning to ride.

4. Riding does not require unusual strength and endurance. The adductor muscles will tire out quickly after a lengthy absence from riding, but that can be prevented by using the aforementioned Groin Stretch and groin-strengthening exercises.

5. There is no cardiorespiratory benefit in horseback riding. It is important that the rider maintain cardiorespiratory fitness through GAF conditioning or some other activity.

Ice Skating The joy of gliding over ice dates back at least to the eighth century, and the best of primitive skates were honed from the bones of cows and other large animals. One of the oldest pictures of skating is a woodcut (dated 1448) of St. Lidwina, the patron saint of skating, who was canonized for the beauty of her spirit. There is an unique exhilaration in ice skating. Today and forever ice skating ranks as one of winter's most pleasurable sports.

For the record there are three different skating categories: figure, hockey, and speed skating. Either figure or hockey skates may be used for recreational skating, but figure skates are preferable because you can do more with them. After all, once your hockey-playing days are over and after Eric Heiden's performance in the 1980 Winter Olympics, you may want to learn something more than starting, stopping, and skating in circles.

BODY PARTS

The key body parts are the legs—from the thighs to the feet, especially the ankles. The most common injuries are pulled hamstrings, Achilles tendinitis, and, for the beginner, sore ankles. In addition, falling accounts for bumps, bruises, and an occasional broken bone. Beginning skaters suffer more often when taking a spill because they have not learned how to fall.

Most of the falls are backward, caused by the feet getting too far in front of the body's center of gravity. The beginner must learn to go with the fall to recover balance and not stick out an arm in anticipation of the fall. The only part of the body that must be protected from a backward fall is the head. Tuck your chin into your chest, and protect the back of the head with your hands.

CONDITIONING

1. General conditioning should be at GAF Level II. Exercises within that program will help prevent pulled hamstrings, Achilles tendinitis and sore ankles—if ice skates fit properly and are laced properly. Give special attention to the warm-up/flexibility and cool-down exercises. The cardiorespiratory conditioning in Extra Edge is also recommended.

2. Specific conditioning is unnecessary if the skater continues with GAF Level II. However, one special exercise to stretch the hip flexors is useful.

HIP FLEXOR STRETCH

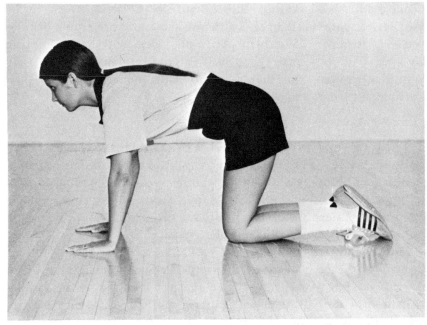

STARTING POSITION

COUNT 1 AND COUNT 2

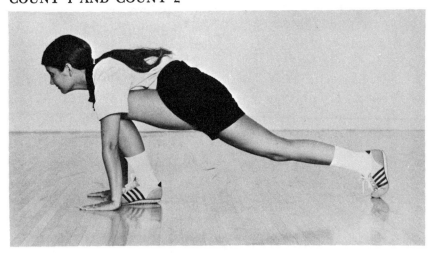

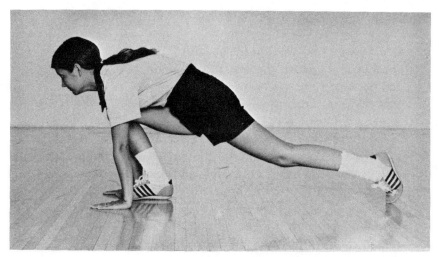

COUNT 3 AND COUNT 4

RETURN TO STARTING
    POSITION

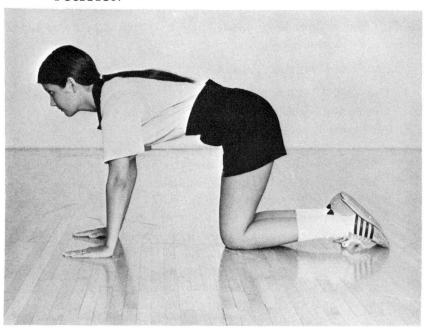

Hip Flexor Stretch

Starting Position: Get down on your hands and knees with your hands separated to shoulder width.

Action: Count 1: Move the left foot forward between your hands. At the same time extend the right foot back with toes in a pushing position. During this action the left heel must touch the floor.

Count 2: Straighten the right leg, and push off the right toe, allowing the body weight to shift forward until the stretch is felt in the hip muscles. Hold for 15 seconds.

Count 3: Reverse the positions of the feet.

Count 4: Straighten the left leg, and push off the left toe, allowing the body weight to shift forward until the stretch is felt in the hip muscles. Hold for 15 seconds.

Cadence: Very slow.

Progression: Start with 5 repetitions, holding each stretch for 15 seconds, and gradually increase to 10 repetitions with 30-second stretches.

3. Preactivity Warm-up: Before putting on your ice skates, perform the warm-up and flexibility exercises from GAF Level II and the Hip Flexor Stretch exercise. These exercises should also be repeated after skating.

HEALTH AND FITNESS ANALYSIS

1. The average skater who weighs 117 pounds will burn about 264 calories per hour; the 150-pound skater, 348 calories.

2. Ice skating is classified as a moderate-activity sport.

3. Children may learn to skate after their fourth birthday or when they can overcome the fear of falling. One is never too old to learn to ice skate if there is adequate coordination and confidence. Only the fear of falling keeps older people from ice skating.

4. Ice skating is enjoyable when there is sufficient strength and endurance in the legs. This can be developed by running.

5. Ice skating is a good cardiorespiratory activity because it requires the use of the legs' large muscles, which in turn pump up the blood. However, ice skating ranks well behind running, swimming, and bicycling as a cardiorespiratory conditioner.

Roller Skating See "Ice Skating" (page 290). All the conditioning information applies to roller skating. The big advantage of roller skating over ice skating is that you do not have to wait until water or hell freezes over to skate. Furthermore, with the introduction of wide polyurethane wheels, skating on blacktop is very satisfactory. However, be alert for gravel, wet surfaces, and pedestrians.

Running/Jogging Running has become a multimillion-dollar industry. It has been made to appear complex, profound, and often ridiculous. Runners talk of having highs and lows and religious experiences. A chic couple spends $300 for running shoes, three how-to-run books, and chic white running suits to run around a drab city block for thirty minutes.

What's happened to the national intelligence? Wasn't running once as simple as walking?

This brief entry proposes to tell you everything that you need to know about running and nothing more.

The running weekender is worrisome. Despite all the books, many runners aren't properly prepared, and as a result, injuries are common. Another disturbing factor is that most runners do nothing else to stay fit. Although cardiorespiratory conditioning is very important, it is not all-important. If you only run, the muscle tone falls off and posture suffers in later years. The runner may have a healthy heart and lungs, but the skeletal muscles, especially the antigravity muscles, fail. This leads to severe structural problems such as low-back pain, which leads to inactivity—and thus a loss of cardiorespiratory fitness.

Runners must have a balanced conditioning program in order to maintain lifetime normal function.

BODY PARTS

The runner's most important body parts are those of the lower body—from the trunk down to the lower extremities. Some runners also complain that the upper torso, specifically the deltoids and trapezius muscles, also groans excessively when they run, especially over long distances.

Because running itself is so specific, injuries occur specifically to the feet, ankles, Achilles tendons, shins, knees, hamstrings, quadriceps, and low back. Most of these injuries are common to other sports activities; that is why weekend runners should think of themselves not as gurus, but as athletes. The most casual weekend runner is well served by reading Part IV, "Body Parts: Their Care and Maintenance." For example, correcting a problem as simple as pronation will promote running performance and prevent pain and injury.

The capacity of the heart to sustain a person during a run or any other vigorous activity is a nagging concern. From time to time, we hear about someone suffering a heart attack during or after exercising. This may occur because the person was not paying attention to the body's alarm system.

Whenever you are exercising, especially if you are over age 35, you should heed certain body signals:

> A heavy pressure in your chest or the feeling of tightness in the chest's center.
> Stiffness in your diaphragm or throat that makes breathing difficult.
> Extreme or persistent pains in the arms, chest, upper abdomen, head, ears, or neck.

Any one of the above symptoms is a signal to stop exercising immediately and warrants a prompt trip to your physician, preferably a cardiologist who will schedule an exercise stress test.

Generally, if you pass a good stress test, you may assume that your heart is healthy and efficient for your age-group. Because no stress test is 100 percent accurate, you should ask the cardiologist to explain the accuracy of the particular protocol used in the test. Furthermore, the cardiologist should be able to tell you if there must be any boundaries to the level of your exercise, whether the activity is running or any other sport.

The above said, you should know that you cannot hurt a healthy heart. In fact, vigorous activities at a level appropriate for your age-group will improve overall cardiovascular efficiency.

CONDITIONING

1. General Athletic Fitness. Running rates as a heavy activity specifically in the context of cardiorespiratory fitness. If you wish to develop your running or run competitively, you must run more than

is required at any level in GAF conditioning, just as the tennis player must play more tennis in order to sharpen the necessary skills.

The GAF conditioning at either Level II or Level III is adequate for the development of overall strength and endurance. The GAF program should be followed at least three times a week, on alternate days, when you are not running, and no fewer than two days. However, on days when you are only running, you should do the GAF warm-up and cool-down exercises before and after the run. Also, on days when you are doing only GAF, you should do everything, including the Extra Edge program.

2. Specific Athletic Fitness. Specific conditioning for the runner is designed to prevent injuries and improve efficiency. The more efficiently you run, the less energy used and the longer stored energy will last. You can run longer and faster.

Specific flexibility exercises for the runner include:

a. Achilles Stretch—GAF flexibility exercise 1, page 98.

b. Hamstring Stretch—GAF flexibility exercises 2, 3, 4, pages 100–105.

c. Quadriceps/Iliopsoas Stretch—GAF flexibility exercise 5, page 106.

d. Groin Stretch—GAF flexibility exercise 6, page 108.

e. Feet Over—GAF flexibility exercise 8, page 112.

f. Foot and Ankle Stretch—GAF flexibility exercise 7, page 110.

Two other important exercises are the Bent-Knee Sit-ups (see page 160) and the shin strengthener or toe lift exercise (see Elevated Toe Raises on page 152).

3. Preactivity Warm-up/Cool-down: If you watch Olympic-caliber runners prepare for competition, you come to see that it takes longer to warm up than to run the race. For the weekender, the warm-up is more important. It is estimated that about 50 percent of running injuries could be prevented by proper warm-up.

You should think of the body's warm-up being similar to warming up a car engine in the winter. At first it is sluggish. Then it gradually begins running smoothly. If you pull out of the garage too soon, the car stalls. Similarly, you will see runners lace on their running shoes and go off at a brisk pace only to stop, sit down and remove their shoes. As with the car engine, the colder it is or the longer the body has been out of use, the longer the warm-up must be.

The warm-up for the experienced runner always begins with stretching exercises, followed by an easy jog. The stretching exercises should be those noted above and any others that you favor. Ten to fifteen minutes are not too much time to spend warming up. The minimum time should be six to eight minutes. Start off with a slow jog or a walk before you pick up your running pace.

When the run is over, cool down slowly. Jog slowly, then walk, and when you have stopped, go through the stretch exercises again.

HEALTH AND FITNESS ANALYSIS

1. A person who weighs 117 pounds and runs on a flat surface at an 8-minute-per-mile pace will burn about 680 calories per hour. The faster you run, the higher the energy expenditure. If you run at a 7-minute-per-mile pace, you will expend an additional 60 to 70 calories.

A 150-pound person burns about 850 calories per hour on a flat run at 8 minutes per mile. A minute faster will expend an additional 90 to 100 calories.

2. Running is classified as a heavy activity only in the legs and cardiovascular system.

3. Any age-group may participate. Older people who have been sedentary for long periods require more time to become comfortable in running. They should begin with slow walking and then gradually progress through brisk walking and slow jogging before running.

4. Because running affects only the lower extremities, it is strongly recommended that you continue GAF Level II or Level III on non-running days to maintain the muscle tone of the upper body.

5. Running is the second best exercise to develop cardiorespiratory fitness for the average person. The best substitutes for running are swimming and bicycling, either stationary or road. The best CR conditioning is found in cross-country skiing if you have the equipment and snow.

Snow Skiing, Cross Country, Downhill   In the 1970's snow skiing became firmly established as a major recreational sport. Downhill skiing continues to be popular, and cross-country skiing is growing at a phenomenal rate. Both deserve to be popular, but they are worlds apart in many ways.

Many people are priced out of downhill skiing. Expenses include lift fees, travel, restaurants, housing, and costly equipment. In downhill, the chances of injury are higher, although many of these accidents may be prevented with preconditioning. Ski slopes are usually crowded, and that means waiting in long lines to use the lifts. Still, if it's affordable, the exhilaration in racing a hill is worth every penny.

Cross-country equipment costs less. The chances of injury are very low. There are no ski fees, no need to travel long distances. You can backpack a picnic lunch, ski in a city park, or, if you live near fields and woods, start out of your backyard. Cross-country is simply skiing the available terrain. It lacks the risk and excitement of speed but is invigorating and has its own exhilaration. There are no crowds—no one but you and your companions touring in the silent, secret world of snow. And it's a helluva workout.

BODY PARTS

Both downhill and cross-country skiing requires strong, flexible leg muscles—especially the quadriceps, hamstrings, and groin muscles of the thighs, the Achilles tendons, and the gastrocnemius of the calves. The trunk muscles, including the back and abdominals, must be strong. In addition, cross-country skiers must have reliable strength and endurance in their arms and shoulder-girdle muscles.

Cardiorespiratory conditioning is important for both kinds of skiing, but for the cross-country skier it is imperative. The average downhill weekender skis in short stretches and under fairly controlled conditions. The demand on the CR system is limited. However, cross-country skiing, even at the recreational level, ranks with running and swimming as a CR activity. Although the beginning cross-country skier has the option of starting off easy, a great proportion of the body's muscle mass is required to perform heavy exertion for extended periods.

The knee is most frequently injured in skiing. However, there are also fractures of the arms and legs; sprained ankles, knees, and wrists; and dislocated shoulders. Most injuries are caused by falls. A high percentage of falls occur on the first downhill run—usually as a result of inadequate warm-up or on the last run of the day because of fatigue, a lack of proper conditioning.

1. General Athletic Fitness. Cross-country rates as a heavy activity. All cross-country skiers, especially beginners, should work at GAF Level III. Once the beginner has learned the rudimentary skills of cross-country skiing and goes out to tour the countryside, he wants to be certain that he has the stamina to get home.

Downhill skiing is not as demanding at the recreational level. Most of the downhiller's time is spent in waiting (and resting) in the lift line. GAF Level II is adequate for most downhill skiers, although the accomplished and competitive skier should work out at Level III. However, and this is important, proper conditioning is critical to all skiers to prevent injury.

2. Specific Athletic Fitness. If you are a novice or intermediate skier, work at GAF Level II at least two times a week. On alternate days, use the following exercises:

    a. GAF flexibility exercises 1, 2, 5, 6, 7, and 9 on pages 98, 100, 106, 108, 110, 114.

    b. Calisthenics.

        (1) *High Jumper* (see page 169).

        (2) *Half Squat* (see page 132).

        (3) *Kangaroo Hop* (see page 301).

KANGAROO HOP

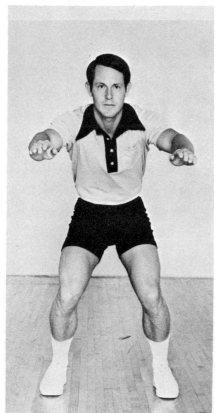

STARTING POSITION

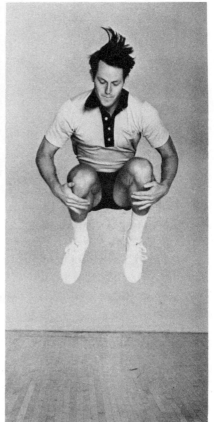

COUNT 1

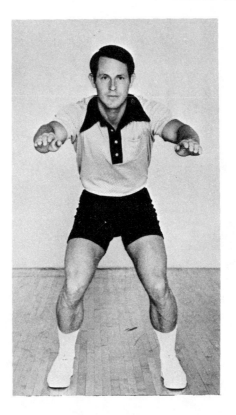

COUNT 2

Starting Position: Stand straight with arms raised in a forward po-
    sition at shoulder height. Feet should be parallel and about
    shoulder width apart, knees slightly flexed.
Action: Count 1: Jump, attempting to bring your knees to your
    chest.
    Count 2: Return to starting position.
Cadence: Moderate to fast.
Progression: Begin with 5 repetitions, and gradually increase to 12
    repetitions.

c. Cardiorespiratory Conditioning. Running is an excellent conditioner. The minimum should be the Extra Edge recommendation
at your GAF level. If snow makes running impossible, jumping rope
is an excellent substitute. Begin with 60 jumps per minute for 2
minutes, and gradually increase to 80 to 100 jumps per minute for
10 minutes. (See page 303.)

JUMPING ROPE

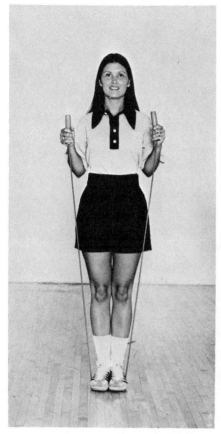

CHECKING PROPER
LENGTH FOR
JUMPING ROPE

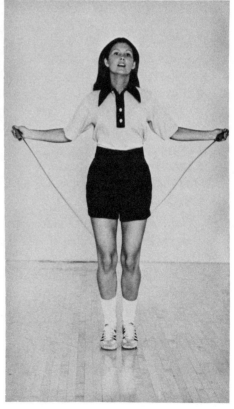

BOXER-STYLE
JUMPING

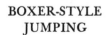

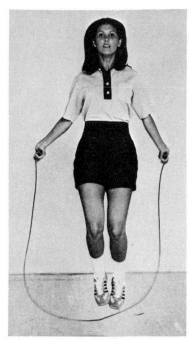

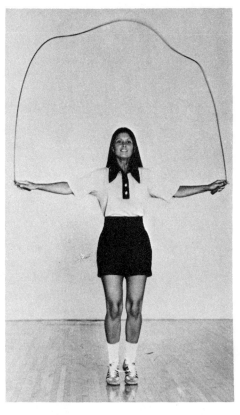

ROPE PASSES UNDER
BOTH FEET AT THE
SAME TIME.

HANDS STAY AT THE
SAME LEVEL WHILE
TURNING THE ROPE.

The cross-country skier must work on developing muscular strength and endurance in the legs, arms, and shoulder girdle and CR fitness. Work with the GAF Level III program at least two times a week. On alternate days use the following exercises at least three times a week:

    a. GAF flexibility exercises 1, 2, 4, 6, 7, and 10 on pages 98–101, 104, 108–111, 115.

    b. Calisthenics.

        (1) *Half Squat* (see page 132).

        (2) *Mountain Climber* (see page 305).

MOUNTAIN CLIMBER

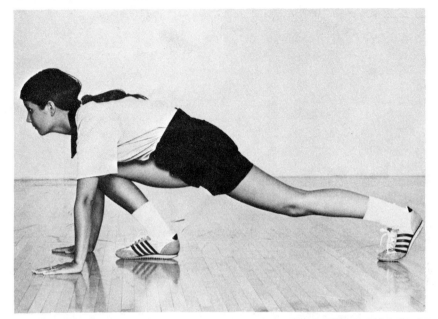

STARTING POSITION

COUNT 1

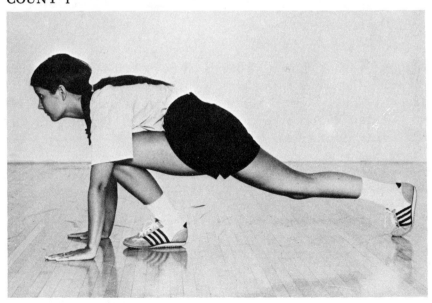

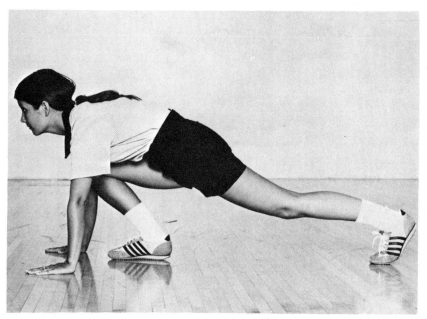

COUNT 2

Starting Position: Squat with hands on floor. Left leg extended to rear. Right knee is inside the right elbow.

Action: Count 1: Reverse position of feet simultanteously.

Count 2: Again reverse position of feet, returning to the starting position.

Cadence: Start at moderate pace. Switch to fast pace.

Progression: Begin by doing 12 repetitions, and gradually increase to 20 repetitions.

(3) *Wall Sit* (see page 307).

WALL SIT

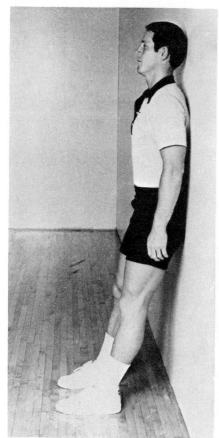

STARTING
POSITION

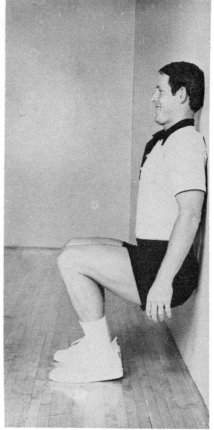

COUNT 1

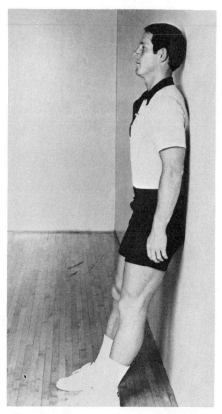

COUNT 2

Starting Position: Stand about one step away from a solid wall, feet
shoulder width apart, back toward wall.
Action: Count 1: Lean backward until your shoulders touch the
wall. Rest the whole of your backside on the wall, and then
slide down until you are in a sitting position. You should then
be supporting your weight with your back and feet. Adjust
your feet until your calves are parallel to the wall. Hold this
position for the prescribed count.
     Count 2: Return to the starting position.
Cadence: Slow.
Progression: Begin by holding the sitting position for 15 seconds,
and repeat for 4 repetitions. Gradually increase to hold for 1
minute, and repeat for 4 repetitions.

c. Cardiorespiratory Conditioning. As a minimum use the Extra
Edge of GAF Level III. You may use rope jumping as a substitute.
Begin jumping with 60 jumps per minute for 3 minutes. Gradually
increase until you are jumping 80 to 100 jumps per minute for
14 minutes.

HEALTH AND FITNESS ANALYSIS

1. A 117-pound downhill skier will burn about 450 calories per hour; a 150-pound downhill skier, about 590 calories per hour during normal recreational skiing. Downhill skiers who are racing should increase these figures by about 60 percent.

A 117-pound cross-country skier will burn about 550 calories per hour; a 150-pound cross-country skier, about 710 calories when skiing on level ground. These figures should be doubled when you are competing on mixed terrain.

2. Downhill skiing by the typical weekend skier is a moderate activity. Cross-country skiing is a heavy activity.

3. Downhill skiing should be learned before the age of 40 unless you are in top physical condition and very active in other sports. There's no doubt that experienced skiers can stay active into their fifties and sixties. However, once you are into your fifties, have an exercise stress test, and consider cross-country skiing, where the chances of accidents are reduced. Also, a partner is strongly recommended for cross-country skiing. The 50-year-old man or woman who has not been athletically active should not take up downhill skiing.

4. Downhill and cross-country skiing require good muscular strength and endurance in the lower body. In addition, cross-country requires strength and endurance in the arm and shoulder-girdle area.

5. Cross-country requires and helps develop extremely high cardiorespiratory fitness. Some of the top competitive cross-country skiers have been reported to have the best CR fitness in the world of sports. Although the recreational downhill skier does not need an extreme level of CR fitness, above-average CR fitness will assure a more enjoyable experience and reduce the chances of accidents at the end of the day. For competitive downhill skiers, CR conditioning should be as high as time will permit.

Weight Lifting Weight lifting is usually thought to attract only a select group—people who are interested in a "body beautiful" and those who compete in Olympic-style weight lifting. However, in recent years some weekenders have been using weight lifting, or weight training, as a practical means of developing muscle groups that have been largely neglected. Some of the weekenders include women, who have learned that weights do not develop gross "masculine" muscles. Some are Hollywood women who depend on weights to maintain spectacular bodies.

Unfortunately many people oversimplify weight lifting. They believe that training is merely a matter of progressing from one weight to another that is heavier. Sporting goods stores promote this misunderstanding with weight lifting sets for children and adults. Some of these products come with instructions, but the program is usually primitive in the context of modern sports research.

Today weight lifting is a very specialized activity that requires the supervision of an expert who may be available at a Y or reputable health club. If you shop around, you discover that there is a variety of specialized equipment that functions differently and employs different principles. They include:

FREE WEIGHTS

These are the classic barbells and dumbbells. This equipment builds strength, but the exercises must be appropriate to the muscle group and performed correctly. Otherwise, you lose flexibility and become muscle-bound. The advantage in free weight training is that you are using the same kind of equipment that is used in local, national, and international competition, either power lifting or Olympic lifting.

Power lifting consists of three exercises: the Squat, the Bench Press, and the Dead Lift.

1. The Squat requires that the athlete start in a standing position with the barbell held behind the head and across the shoulder. The lifter must then perform a full squat—until the midline of the thighs is below an imaginary plane that passes through the knees and is parallel to the floor. The lifter must then rise and return to the starting position.

2. In the Bench Press the lifter lies on a bench with his face upward. The barbell is held with fully outstretched arms directly above the chest. The barbell is lowered to the chest. A pause of a second is allowed, and the barbell is raised again until the arms are fully extended.

3. The Dead Lift requires raising the barbell from the floor until

the lifter is completely erect. The weight is held with arms fully extended downward.

The Olympic Lifts, so named because they are used at the Olympic Games, are performed much more rapidly than power lifting.

1. In the Snatch, the barbell is lifted from the floor overhead with arms fully extended in one movement in order to take advantage of the momentum once the lifter gets the weight moving.

2. The Clean and Jerk has two movements. In the clean movement, the weight is lifted from the floor to the shoulders just under the chin. In the jerk movement, the weight is raised overhead with the arms fully extended.

Although these lifts, power and Olympic, are very simple, the weekender should be warned that training is very specific. The results are too specialized to be useful in other sports. The great majority of weekenders are interested not in lifting strength, but in functional strength that can be used in recreational competition. Free weights can be used to help functional strength, but the training must have the supervision of a competent instructor.

NAUTILUS EQUIPMENT

The Nautilus system is a series of machines, each designed to strengthen a specific muscle or major muscle group. The key to this equipment is a cam, devised to provide variable resistance throughout the full range of motion of the joint as the exercise is performed. The variable resistance compensates for stress differences during the exercise and thus assures that the muscle group is being equally stressed throughout the full range of motion.

The Nautilus system has several major advantages. It is effective and safe, develops strength throughout the full range of motion, and improves the flexibility of the body parts that are exercised. You work through a variety of machines, which helps avoid boredom, and it is boredom that causes most people to drop out of a conditioning program.

Nautilus equipment is very expensive but available in a number of clubs throughout the country.

THE UNIVERSAL GYM

This is a versatile "small weight" machine that duplicates most of the barbell exercises. The equipment is appropriately popular at the high school level for a number of reasons. It eliminates many of the safety hazards that exist in using barbells, it requires limited floor space, weights are increased or decreased simply, safely, and with ease, and it requires less exercise time than working with barbells. The newest Universal Gym offers variable resistance in an attempt to accommodate the changes in mechanical advantage as the weight is raised and lowered.

The weekender is apt to find the Universal Gym in Ys, local high schools, and health clubs. The machines are effective in building strength when properly used in a well-designed program. However, the Universal Gym lacks the flexibility improvement built into the Nautilus. The weekender who uses the Universal Gym or free weights should request the instructor to advise him in the correct use in order to maintain and increase flexibility.

Chapter 18

Dual/Court Sports

Badminton (M)
Handball (H)
Paddle Tennis (M/H)
Platform Tennis (M)
Racquetball/Paddle Ball (H)
Squash (H)
Tennis (M/H)

The dual/court classification, although an invention of the authors, is not an arbitrary term. A dual, or two-person, sports tells us something about the size of a game. We know at once that it won't be played on a football or baseball field. Through centuries of usage we also know that "court" suggests a limited area that is usually enclosed.

Game area is a result of competitive experience. Youngsters sense this when playing one-on-one basketball and use less than a fifth of the court. When we go from tennis doubles to singles, eliminating the alleys, the playing area loses 702 square feet, a 25 percent reduction in the size of the court.

To an inexperienced observer, court games appear to accommodate the players, making it easier to reach the ball. In fact, the smaller the court, the more quickly the ball is returned, the faster the ball moves, and the greater the need for fast reaction. Small court games demand a high degree of mental and physical agility, speed, coordination, and constant alertness, which in turn demands an extra edge of muscular and mental endurance. All dual/court sports have the above in common, whether you whack the ball with wood or your hands.

In this category we will cover eight court sports. Some are popular around the world; others enjoy regional popularity. The games differ significantly, but all make similar demands on the specific body parts. For example, the squash forehand differs from the tennis forehand. Each requires different practice to develop coordination, but the biomechanical conditioning is the same.

Important Body Parts in Dual/Court Sports

Although the entire body is called into play, sports research has identified the most important body parts:

—Hands and forearms grip strength is a common, weekender weakness, especially among beginners and most women. Perhaps grip-strength exercises are the most boring because it would appear that few weekenders make an effort to remedy this problem.

—Upper-arm and shoulder-girdle strength and flexibility are important in developing power in our strokes and are also a major factor in preventing tennis elbow.

—The muscles of the stomach and lower back are another factor in developing a power stroke.

—The legs must be strong and flexible to move us around the court and also increase the power of our stroke.

—The cardiorespiratory system must be properly conditioned. If we cannot get adequate amounts of oxygen to the muscles, their strength makes little difference. Dual/court sports require a mix of CR conditioning, which should include some anaerobics (sprints, running upstairs, fast rope jumping) and the aerobic (long, slow workouts.)

The most publicized injury in racquet/paddle sports is the tennis elbow. This injury is described in Part III, "Body Parts." Other injuries include Achilles tendonitis, sprained ankles and knees, pulled hamstrings and groin muscles, and low-back sprains. The conditioning prescribed in this section will give you a great measure of protection.

An unrecognized side effect, pun intended, of racquet sports is posture imbalance because one side of the body is developed more than the other. This can lead to curvature of the spine and eventually to back pain. For that reason the weekender is urged to exercise the entire body by using the General Athletic Fitness. Furthermore, the Specific Athletic Fitness program should be used for both sides of the body. For instance, in developing one's grip and shoulder-girdle strength and flexibility, both hands and both shoulders should be conditioned equally.

Conditioning

1. General Athletic Fitness. The recommended GAF programs for the different dual/court sports are specifically designed for the weekender's level of play. The program also takes into consideration the limited time available to the weekender player.

a. *Badminton.* Although badminton is very demanding when evenly matched opponents compete, GAF Level II is the proper level of conditioning for average singles play. If you are playing at a highly competitive level against highly skilled opponents, you should condition at GAF Level III. This high level of play is more common in England and in some of the southeastern Asian countries, where badminton is usually played indoors to eliminate wind conditions. Finally, if you play doubles most of the time, GAF Level I is adequate.

b. *Handball.* Another demanding sport, handball appears to be slipping in popularity perhaps because of the increasing popularity of racquetball, which uses the same four-wall courts. As a result, handball players are finding that courts are less frequently available. Handball is more of a challenge than racquetball because you must learn to use both hands to control the ball through different spins. General conditioning is recommended at GAF Level III. However, if you regularly play doubles or with an opponent who plays a moderate game, GAF Level II is satisfactory.

c. *Paddle Tennis.* This game enjoys regional popularity. It is played with a short-handled paddle on an undersized court, exactly one-fourth the size of a standard tennis court. The game is easy to learn but, when played at a highly competitive, skilled level, requires GAF Level III conditioning. When it is played as a doubles game, GAF Level II is appropriate.

d. *Platform Tennis.* This game is an intriguing combination of tennis and a wall-court game such as handball or racquetball. The platform court is surrounded by a wire fence, a little like heavy chicken wire. Using a short-handled, large-faced racquet, the ball may be played off the ground or the wall. In doubles, GAF Level II is appropriate. As a singles game, GAF Level III is recommended.

e. **Racquetball and Paddle Ball.** Both games are easy to learn. Both are played on a one-wall, three-wall, or four-wall court. Paddle ball is played with a wood, steel, or plastic paddle; racquetball uses a short strung racquet. Both games are heavy-activity sports, making GAF Level III conditioning appropriate. However, if you are not highly skilled and play "just for the fun of it" against an opponent who shares your attitude, GAF Level II is satisfactory.

f. **Squash.** This four-wall game classifies as a heavy-activity sport that requires quick movements to get to the ball. GAF Level III conditioning is necessary.

g. **Tennis.** Doubles rate as a moderate activity with GAF Level II appropriate. Singles, a heavy activity, call for GAF Level III conditioning.

2. Specific Athletic Fitness. For all dual/court sports, the weekend athlete should schedule the specified GAF programs on two alternate days of a week and the SAF program that follows on other alternate days. On game days use only the warm-up/cool-down sequence. For suggested schedules see pages 141–142.

SAF workout: Two or more days a week, preferably not on consecutive days.

Warm-up: GAF flexibility exercises 1, 2, 6, 8, 9, and 10 on pages 98–101, 108, 112, 115.

Bent-Knee Sit-up (see page 160).

SIDE HOP

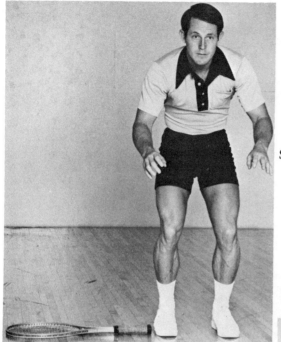

STARTING POSITION

COUNT 1

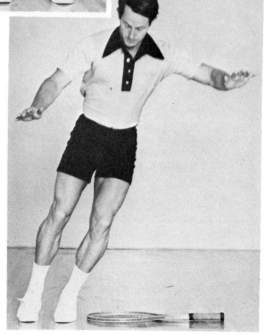

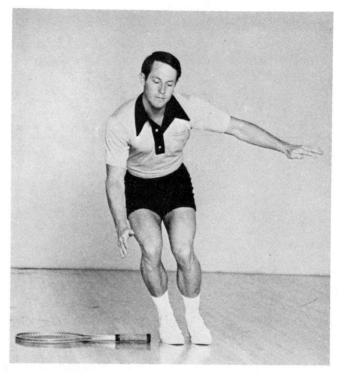

COUNT 2

Side Hop

Starting Position: **Place a towel, shirt, or racquet on the ground
    to the right side of your right foot. Start exercise from a stand-
    ing, upright position.**
Action: Count 1: Jumping simultaneously with both feet, jump
    sideways over the towel.
    Count 2: Jump sideways to the left, and return to the start-
    ing position.
Cadence: Start with a moderate cadence, and increase to a fast
    cadence.
Progression: Begin with 10 repetitions. Increase to 25 repetitions.
    The next time you do this exercise begin by jumping to the
    left.

Mountain Climber (see page 305)

Starting Position: Squat with hands on floor, left leg extended to the rear, right knee inside the right elbow.
Action: Count 1: Reverse position of the feet simultaneously.
    Count 2: Again reverse the position, returning to the starting position.
Cadence: Start moderately, and increase to fast.
Progression: Start with 15 repetitions, and increase to 30.

Push-ups (see page 155)

Progression: Begin with 20 repetitions, and increase to 30 repetitions. Begin the exercise by doing the first five push-ups from the fingertips. Gradually increase fingertip push-ups to 15.

Towel Twist (see Grip Strength exercise on page 355)

Ball Squeeze (see Grip Strength exercise on page 352)
    Note: Handball players may skip the Ball Squeeze. However, the Towel Twist strengthens the muscles (pronators and supinators) that the handball player uses to put spin on a ball.

STAR RUN TEST

The layout of the Star Run Test on the racquetball court is shown in the following diagram:

FRONT WALL

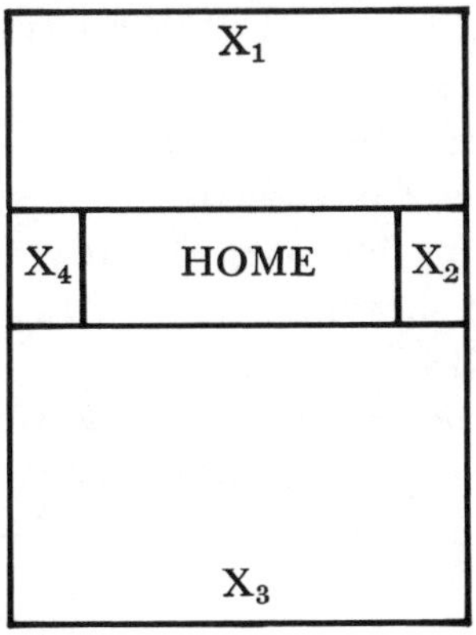

The Star Run test/conditioner is performed as follows: begin at the HOME location, sprint to location X_1; touch the floor just front of where it meets the wall with one hand; sprint back to the HOME location; touch the floor with one hand; sprint to location X_2; again touch the floor with one hand just in front of where it meets the wall; touch; and return to the HOME location. . . . Continue the same pattern—sprinting, touching, sprinting, touching—throughout the 45-second time limit of the test. One point is scored each time the HOME location or any of the four X locations are touched.

The cardiorespiratory conditioning (running, bicycling, swimming) in the GAF program is aerobic. The Star Run Test, illustrated above, is designed to improve your anaerobic conditioning. The Star Run has been developed by Dr. Robert Stauffer, director of research and evaluation of West Point's Department of Physical Education. Dr. Stauffer invented the Star Run as an exercise and test for the classes in racquetball. However, it may also be used for handball and paddle ball and, with slight variations to match the court, for badminton, squash, tennis, platform tennis, and paddle tennis.

If you decide to give the Star Run a try, first warm up properly, and then walk through it several times to learn the pattern. Run the test at quarter speed, then at half speed, and finally at full speed. For conditioning purposes it would be best to schedule the Star Run at the end of your workout so you won't have to do an additional warm-up.

The Star Run progression should be:

a. Run at less than full speed. Rest for two minutes.

b. Repeat.

c. Run at full speed. Rest for four minutes.

d. Run at full speed. Cool down.

As your conditioning improves, you may increase the number of times you run at full speed, or you can reduce the amount of rest time between the full-speed runs.

The object of the rest time is to allow your heart rate to return to near normal. As your conditioning improves, your heart rate will return faster to a near-normal heart rate. However, you should expect to allow a minimum of two minutes' rest between runs.

This is primarily an anaerobic activity, which means that the body cannot meet the total oxygen demands. As a result, an oxygen debt (or shortage) builds within the body. The rest periods are necessary for the cardiorespiratory system to pay back the oxygen debt. Because this is an anaerobic exercise, you may expect to find that the more often you repeat the run, the more difficult it will be to maintain the pace.

Dr. Stauffer uses the scale that follows to grade the cadets. If you play racquetball, handball, or paddle ball, you may want to compare yourself with a cadet.

West Point Racquetball/Handball/Paddle Ball
Star Run Test Rating Scale

Rating	Men Raw Points	Women Raw Points
Excellent (A)	35–37	30–32
Good (B)	32–34	27–29
Average (C)	30–31	25–26
Below Average (D)	28–29	23–24
Failing (F) Or Needs More Work	27 and below	22 and below

3. Warm-ups/Cool-downs, to be used on game days immediately before and after competition.

(a) Begin with a two- or three-minute light jog around the court.

(b) Use GAF flexibility exercise 1 (page 98), stretch out the Achilles tendons; a combination of 2, 3, or 4 (pages 100–105), to stretch out the hamstrings and lower back: 6 to stretch the groin muscles and 8 to stretch the back muscles; 10 can be used with your racquet to loosen the shoulder muscles.

(c) Before taking off your racquet cover, practiec some dummy swings before hitting a ball. The cover will offer some resistance and make your racquet feel a little lighter when it comes off.

After competition, cool off with a brief, slow jog and repeat the flexibility exercises.

Health and Fitness

Badminton

1. A 117-pound person playing recreational badminton will burn about 264 calories per hour; a 150-pound person, 336 calories. In competitive badminton, a 117-pound person will burn about 460 calories per hour; a 150-pound person, 595 calories.

2. Recreational badminton rates as a moderate activity. Competitive badminton is a heavy activity.

3. Badminton can be played at any age as a recreational sport. Participants in competitive badminton must be in excellent condition and be able to make quick stops and starts.

4. Badminton requires good strength mainly in the legs and trunk in order to move quickly.

5. A high level of cardiorespiratory fitness is a prime prerequisite in competitive badminton. For the weekend athlete, the level of cardiorespiratory fitness need not be extreme, but it must be adequate—at least at the Extra Edge level of GAF Level II.

Handball

1. A 117-pound person will burn about 485 calories per hour; a 150-pound person, 630 calories.

2. Handball starts as a heavy activity.

3. You will find men playing handball into their sixties. These are men who have been playing consistently for twenty, thirty, forty years. Superior experience gives them the advantage of better placement of the ball, which results in their opponents' doing the heavy running. However, handball should be learned before the mid-forties. From that age on, try racquetball.

4. Handball requires adequate strength in the arms, chest, and shoulders—on both sides of the body—and good strength in the legs and trunk muscles.

5. Cardiorespiratory fitness is important at a high level. The Extra Edge fitness at GAF Level III plus the Star Run drill is adequate.

Paddle Tennis

1. A 117-pound person playing doubles burns about 325 calories per hour; a 150-pound person, 420 calories. A 117-pound person playing singles burns about 460 calories per hour; a 150-pound person, 540 calories.

2. Doubles rates as a moderate activity; singles, heavy.

3. Paddle tennis can be played by most people under the age of 65. However, when over 50, one should be in excellent physical condition and should concentrate on playing doubles. The exception is the person who has been playing regularly prior to the age of 50; if that person is in good health, there is no reason to switch from singles.

4. Paddle tennis requires adequate strength in the upper arms and shoulder girdle, good grip strength, and good strength in the legs and trunk in order to be able to cover the court.

5. Cardiorespiratory fitness is important in singles and to a lesser extent in playing doubles. The Extra Edge level of cardiorespiratory fitness at GAF Level II is adequate for doubles and GAF III for singles.

Platform Tennis   The health and fitness analysis is the same as for paddle tennis (see above).

Racquetball/Paddle Ball

1. A 117-pound person burns about 485 calories per hour; a 150-pound person, 630 calories.

2. Racquetball and paddle ball are classified as heavy activity sports.

3. Both games can be played at almost any age when opponents are evenly matched. Good physical condition is a prerequisite.

4. Both require adequate strength in the upper arms and shoulder girdle, good grip strength, and good strength in the legs and trunk in order to be able to cover the court adequately.

5. High levels of cardiorespiratory fitness are required to play these games. The Extra Edge fitness at GAF Level III should be adequate.

Squash

1. A 117-pound person will burn about 490 calories per hour; a 150-pound person, 640 calories.

2. Squash is a heavy-activity sport.

3. Squash can be played at almost any age by evenly matched opponents. However, it requires quick movements, and this may make the game less enjoyable for the person over 50 who is learning squash. On the other hand, if you have been playing squash for years, there is no reason to stop at age 50.

4. Squash requires good grip, arm, and shoulder girdle strength to hit with power. Good leg strength is necessary in order to cover the court.

5. Cardiorespiratory fitness is very important. Plenty of extra running—both long-distance and sprints—is necessary to play competitively. Squash requires quick stops and starts, meaning that anaerobic conditioning is as important as aerobic. The Star Run is appropriate as an anaerobic conditioner.

Tennis

1. A 117-pound person playing doubles burns about 330 calories per hour; a 150-pound person, 425 calories. A 117-pound person playing singles burns about 465 calories per hour; a 150-pound person, 560 calories.

2. Singles is a heavy activity; doubles, moderate.

3. Tennis can be played at any age. However, from age 54 on, most people should stick to doubles. For the person 54 and over who has been an active tennis player, an occasional singles match with someone your own age and ability is reasonable.

4. Tennis requires good strength and endurance in the grip, arm and shoulder girdle, trunk and leg muscles.

5. Cardiorespiratory fitness is important for all tennis players. The Extra Edge level at GAF Level II is recommended for doubles; GAF Level III, for singles.

Chapter 19

Combative Sports

Fencing (M)
Judo (H)
Karate H)

A complete list of combative sports would include such activities as boxing, wrestling, and kendo, but we will analyze only the three that are most popular with the weekend athlete—fencing, judo, and karate. All three should be put in a correct moral context. Although these skills originated as martial arts, they are practiced today as skilled arts.

The sword ceased being a weapon in the eighteenth century. By the time George Washington proposed a military academy at West Point, such patriots as Aaron Burr and Alexander Hamilton settled questions of honor with dueling pistols. However, fencing, an art that requires agility, dexterity, and grace, continued as an honored sport. (In recognition of the esteem held for fencing, the director of the Academy's Physical Education Department carried the prestigious title Master of Fencing and Master of the Sword until 1958.) Similarly, judo and karate, both Oriental in origin, had their beginnings as offensive and defensive skills but have continued as challenging sports.

At the Academy, cadets are taught that there is a clear distinction between self-defense and the sports. Self-defense and close-quarters-combat courses are taught for what they must be—a mix of boxing, wrestling, judo, karate, and just plain dirty city street fighting. There is nothing sporting about self-defense. Although karate and judo may be some help in learning to defend yourself, these skills are not most effective unless you are a truly experienced expert. For example, a woman cadet is told that if she is being attacked by a rapist, a club is more effective than a hand chop.

As the beginner will learn, judo and karate are very stylistic. In fact, a great deal of time is devoted to learning ritual which in itself has little use if you are attacked on the street.

Fencing, judo, and karate are combative only in origin.

Fencing Fencing is a sport that grew out of swordsmanship. There is no intent in fencing to inflict bodily harm. In fact, minimum equipment includes a padded jacket, a face mask, a padded glove, and a blunted weapon. There are three basic weapons—the foil, the epée, and the saber. The novice starts with the foil. Women use only the foil because it is light and does not require as much arm strength as the other two weapons.

Instruction by a qualified fencing instructor is absolutely essential. Instruction is not readily available except in large metropolitan areas or near universities.

Fencing is a major Olympic sport. Most American fencers learn the sport in college clubs. This late start accounts for Americans not being a significant threat in international competition.

BODY PARTS

In fencing, primary emphasis is on the en garde position, the lunge, and the retreat or recovery from the lunge. This requires muscular strength and endurance of the arms and shoulders, low back, and the legs along with good flexibility in the same areas.

The cardiorespiratory demand is more anaerobic than aerobic. The fencer should work at high-speed interval training but not neglect aerobic training. The GAF program takes both into consideration, and the SAF program gets to the specifics of the arms and legs.

CONDITIONING

1. General Athletic Fitness. Fencing, a moderate activity at the weekend level, requires GAF Level II. The Bend and Reach, Squat Thrust, and Push-Up exercises should be performed rapidly to develop functional muscular strength and endurance conditioning. The run in the Extra Edge develops aerobic conditioning.

2. Specific Athletic Fitness. The fencer's specific conditioning includes exercises to improve flexibility and muscular endurance and strength of the arms, shoulders, and legs.

a. Arm Circles (see page 327).

SAF EXERCISES–FENCING

ARM CIRCLES

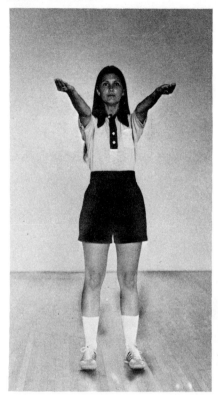

STARTING
POSITION

GRADUALLY

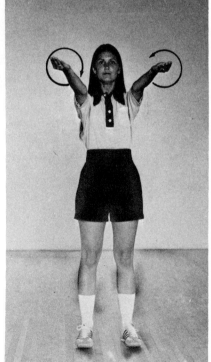

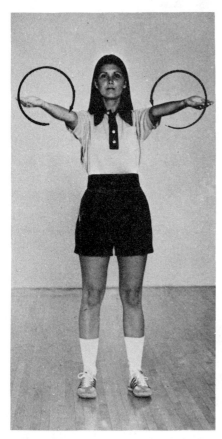

INCREASE

THE SIZE OF THE

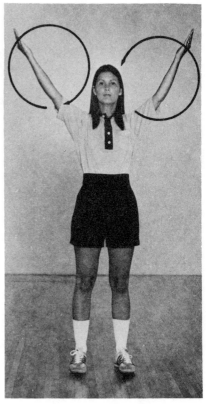

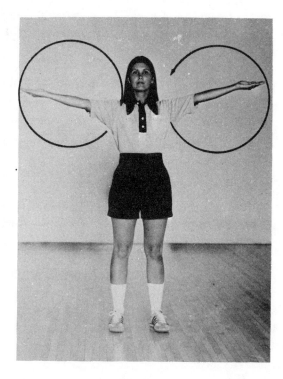

CIRCLES.

Starting Position: Stand with feet separated to shoulder width, head up, buttocks and stomach tucked in, arms extended at shoulder height to the front and parallel to the floor.

Action: Count 1: With palms up, rotate arms to the outside 15 times. Begin with small circles, and gradually increase the circle as large as possible.

Count 2: Drop arms to sides, and relax for a count of 10.

Count 3: Repeat count 1 with rotations in the opposite direction.

Count 4: Drop arms to sides, and relax for a count of 10.

Cadence: Moderate to fast.

Progression: Start with 15 arm circles repeated 5 times. Gradually increase to 30 arm circles for 10 repetitions.

b. Step-ups (see GAF Level III, page 166). Begin with 25 repetitions at a fast cadence, and increase to 50 repetitions at a fast cadence.

c. High Jumper (see GAF Level III, page 169). Begin with 25 repetitions at a fast cadence, and gradually increase to 50 repetitions at a fast cadence.

d. Before and after doing the above exercise, perform the following GAF flexibility exercises: 5, 6, 8, and 9, pages 106, 108, 112, 114.

3. Preactivity Warm-up/Cool-down. On days when you will be fencing in practice, work through the entire SAF program. You may also include some of the GAF Level II exercises, especially the stretchers.

On days when you compete, limit your pre-event workout to the flexibility exercises. You may do all those in GAF Level II plus those in SAF. As a minimum you should do flexibility exercises 1, 3, 5, 6, 7, 8, and 9. Repeat these after competition to cool down.

HEALTH AND FITNESS ANALYSIS

1. A 117-pound person will burn 250 calories; a 150-pound person, 310 calories. However, when expert fencers compete vigorously, the calorie output nearly doubles.

2. At the weekend level, fencing classifies as a moderate-activity sport. Actually very few weekend fencers have the expertise to compete at a high-activity rate.

3. People who fence regularly can continue until almost any age. However, people who have been inactive will find learning fencing difficult after age 40 because of the loss of flexibility and balance. That loss, by the way, is the result of inactivity, not aging. Still, it's conceivable that if you have the patience, you can regain most of the flexibility that you have let slip away.

4. Obviously flexibility and muscular strength and endurance are necessary in the legs, arms, and trunk. However, fencing tends to make greater demands on the dominant side of the body. In order to maintain body balance, every fencer must remember to strengthen and stretch both sides of the body equally.

5. Running and rope skipping are the best methods for developing cardiorespiratory fitness. Fencing itself does little to develop the CR system. However, as noted earlier, both aerobic and anaerobic fitness is essential to compete.

Judo   In ancient China, lama monks developed jujitsu to defend themselves against highway bandits. About the same time the samurai were also developing a weaponless form of combat in Japan. During the 1600's Japanese travelers to the mainland studied the lamas' techniques. This enabled the samurai to add more than 300 throws and holds. For centuries jujitsu was secretly taught to the Japanese nobility. With the end of feudalism jujitsu was introduced into Japanese schools and gymnasiums and became a popular sport.

During World War II virtually all the armies of the world introduced jujitsu to combat troops. Jujitsu, now called judo, is so popular throughout the world that it has been recognized as a sport by the Amateur Athletic Union since 1953 and as an Olympic event since 1964. Judo demands the most efficient use of mental and physical energy. Strength and balance are essential components in order to demonstrate superior holding, choking, and throwing techniques. Judo proficiency is rated by colored belts: white for the beginner, followed by three different brown belts as skills improve, with black only for the expert.

BODY PARTS

Judo requires total body conditioning because the important elements are holding and throwing skills along with learning to distribute the force of a fall in order to prevent injury. Strength and flexibility of the arms, shoulders, back, trunk, and legs are mandatory. Beginners shouldn't consider seeking out a competent instructor until they have reached the final state of conditioning in GAF Level III.

CONDITIONING

1. General Athletic Fitness. GAF Level III should be the minimum goal of the competitor. Stretching is vital in order to prevent muscle pulls. The Extra Edge cardiorespiratory conditioning is essential to develop stamina. The running should be supplemented with rope jumping. If you jump rope for 10 minutes at the rate of 100 to 120 jumps per minute, you will earn about the same amount of CR conditioning as a 2-mile run in 16 minutes.

2. Specific Athletic Fitness. Beyond GAF Level III, judo requires specific work on grip strength plus stretching exercises to improve total body flexibility.

Recommended exercises include:

a. Towel Twist (see Grip Strength, page 351).

  b. Ball Squeeze (see Grip Strength, page 352).

  c. GAF flexibility exercises 1 through 10 (pages 98–117).

  d. Cardiorespiratory condition per instructions Extra Edge, GAF Level III (page 159), or skip rope for 10 minutes at 100 to 120 jumps per minute.

  3. Precompetition Warm-up/Cool-down. On days that you will be competing in practice, perform all exercises listed under SAF. For real competition, plan a 30-minute warm-up using all the flexibility exercises in the GAF flexibility section. At the least, perform 1, 2–5, 6–8 and 10.

HEALTH AND FITNESS ANALYSIS

  1. A 117-pound person will burn about 600 calories per hour during vigorous judo practice or competition; a 150-pound person, 780 calories.

  2. Judo rates as a heavy-activity sport. Participants must be well trained and conditioned to avoid serious injury.

  3. Judo is for the young. However, if judo is learned as a young person, competition may continue, on a very controlled basis, into the forties. No one should try to learn the formal method of judo after age 30. On the other hand, a child of 10 is not too young to learn. As a general rule, the younger you are, the sooner you will become conditioned and develop enough skill to compete.

  4. Total body muscular strength and endurance are necessary to compete successfully. Grip strength, arms and shoulders, trunk, and legs must all be well conditioned. Flexibility is important to prevent injuries.

  5. Running and rope jumping are recommended in developing cardiorespiratory fitness for judo. Because of short periods of vigorous activity, judo is primarily an anaerobic activity. However, aerobic conditioning is essential as a base for building anaerobic fitness.

  Karate Like judo, karate originated in China and eventually traveled to Korea and Okinawa. In the 1900's an Okinawan teacher introduced karate techniques to Japan and established what we know as modern karate.

  There are several different styles of karate, all developed by different Oriental teachers. The Okinawan and Korean styles tend to emphasize force and strength. The Japanese styles, most commonly used in competition, emphasize speed and agility.

In competition, physical contact is strictly limited and not required for scoring. Blows and kicks are "pulled" before contact. Only light contact is permitted on the body, and very light contact on the face and head. Excessive physical contact results in disqualification. Karate participants are ranked according to belt color when competing. Ten belt ranks are designated in colors—white, yellow, green, brown—and ten in black.

BODY PARTS

Karate requires superb conditioning of the total body. The West Point cadet karate team is one of our best-conditioned teams. To develop strength, cadets work with weights and then practice blows and kicks against dummies and striking boards. Before practice, the team spends 30 to 45 minutes in stretching exercises to guarantee flexibility. Balance is developed through hours of practice. Speed and agility are developed with increasing strength and hours of practice. Karate demands hard work and hours of practice under excellent coaching to develop the needed skills. Obviously GAF Level III must be your minimum goal.

CONDITIONING

1. General Athletic Fitness. As a very heavy activity, karate requires GAF Level III conditioning plus emphasis on flexibility exercises and cardiorespiratory conditioning for stamina. CR conditioning should include Extra Edge running or rope jumping for a minimum of 10 minutes at 100 to 120 jumps per minute.

2. Specific Athletic Fitness. Karate skills are very specific and are in themselves conditioning drills that are necessary to develop the proper fitness. However, the weekend karate participant should work on all the GAF flexibility exercises (pages 98–117), between practice session.

In addition, you will learn other exercises during instruction.

3. Precompetition Warm-up/Cool-down. These exercises are best learned from a qualified karate instructor.

HEALTH AND FITNESS ANALYSIS

1. A 117-pound person will burn about 600 calories per hour

during vigorous competition or practice; a 150-pound person, 780 calories.

2. Karate rates as a heavy-activity sport. Total body conditioning, especially flexibility, is extremely important to prevent injuries and to learn the necessary skills.

3. Like judo, karate is for the young in body. Children may learn the skills requiring flexibility and balance but should not practice some other skills during prepuberty, such as striking skills against a hard target. However, kicks at soft targets are not a problem. If a young adult continues to work out regularly, controlled competition can continue into the forties. However, if you were to lay off for several years, you would have to spend as much time as any novice in reconditioning yourself. In karate, knowledge and past experience are not substitutes for fitness. Beginners should seek out a qualified instructor and learn the skills thoroughly before engaging in competition.

4. High-level karate requires excellent flexibility and balance as well as excellent muscular strength and endurance throughout the body.

5. Karate is primarily anaerobic, but this does not lessen the importance of aerobic conditioning. Running and rope jumping are the best methods of developing cardiorespiratory fitness.

Chapter 20

Team Sports

Baseball/Softball (M)
Basketball (H)
Soccer (H)
Touch/Flag Football (H)
Volleyball (M)

If there is such a thing as pure pleasure in sports competition, the weekend athlete gets more of it than the professional, Olympic, college, or even high school athlete. All but the weekender are looking for something extra—scholarships and publicity, contracts and publicity, bonuses and publicity, gold medals and publicity, and, of course, the ultimate recognition, TV commercials. These rewards are compatible with the work and effort required in high-level competition, and there's nothing new about this practice.* However, the truly human rewards of sports competition are enjoyed only by the weekender, and this is especially true of the camaraderie, shared exultation, and unit esprit of team sports.

Throughout the country we have "scheduled games" being played by the working population—among businessmen, doctors, lawyers,

* For the record, the heaping of rewards and publicity on athletes is as old as the history of sports. Conventional wisdom has it that we have compromised sports today and that we should look back at the ancient Greek example of honoring the victor only with an olive crown. In fact, Greek athletes received far more than garlands of wild olive and far more than any modern-day Olympic winner or MVP. Greek athletes were overwhelmed with gifts and favors that ranged from costly gold crowns and jewelry to special privileges, including the attendance of a surrogate goddess. And publicity? Sculptors carved statues of winners for public adulation, and the great poets composed songs in their praise. The athlete was more of a hero, more honored than philosophers, scientists, artists, generals, and political leaders. By comparison, twentieth-century rewards are very modest.

teachers, broadcaster, government bureaucrats, church club members, and industrial employees. The games are scheduled after work and on weekends. They are played for pleasure but are also valuable in developing community and company morale. Team members learn to cooperate for the common goal and subordinate personal instincts for the good of the team. Some sociologists note with regret that most women lack this important experience.

Unfortunately weekenders are poorly prepared for team competition. As a result, sprains, strains and injuries are common. Of course, the joy of competition cannot be fully experienced if you are rusty and short of vigor. The following is a guideline to a level of conditioning commensurate with the needs of the after-hours team player.

Baseball/Softball   The conditioning for baseball and softball is similar, although the harder, smaller, and faster baseball calls for more agility and alertness. However, both are slow games with occasional intensive activity for very brief periods, usually less than thirty seconds. Often the maximum workout is the trot from the outfield to the dugout.

The nature of baseball and softball, the lack of continuous activity, results in many, if not most, ballplayers' being in questionable physical condition, and this includes the professionals. So injuries occur frequently and hurt a team. Too often, as we know, the benching of only one player may shatter a winning streak and lose a pennant.

There is a lot of room for improvement in the physical conditioning of ballplayers at all levels of competition. Although baseball may appear to be the most peaceful and least demanding of games, in one moment of activity the player may have to move quickly and intensely with the whole of the body, and its parts must be ready.

BODY PARTS

Baseball and softball require running, sprinting, throwing, catching, and hitting. All these actions demand strength and flexibility of the arms and shoulder girdle, the trunk and legs. Injuries are normally caused by inadequate strengthening and stretching of the muscles. Elbow and shoulder injuries have terminated many professional careers. The lack of flexibility or inadequate warm-up is the cause of pulled hamstrings and groin muscles. Insufficient grip strength diminishes the batter's power.

CONDITIONING

1. General Athletic Fitness. Both sports rate as moderate activities. The whole of the GAF Level II program, including the cardiorespiratory conditioning in Extra Edge, is recommended for the weekender who wants to enjoy the game fully.

2. Specific Athletic Fitness. There are several simple and specific exercises that will improve the weekender's game and go far toward preventing injuries. These should be performed in addition to the GAF Level II program, although you may choose to do the SAF workout on alternate days.

    a. *Towel Twist* (see Grip Strength, page 355).

    b. *Ball Squeeze* (see Grip Strength, page 352).

    c. *Sprinting.* Anaerobic exercise is a specific conditioner for baseball and softball. (You will get your aerobic conditioning in the slower, longer distances that are part of the GAF program.)

Sprinting exercises begin with a warm-up with some stretching exercises and light jogging. The same exercises are recommended to warm up for running (see page 297). After the warm-up perform the following sets:

Set I. Sprint at half speed: 3 x 50 yards with 10-second rest between sprints.

Set II: Sprint at three-quarters speed: 3 x 50 yards with 10-second rest between sprints.

Set III. Sprint at full speed: 3 x 40 yards with 10-second rest between sprints.

Rest for 30 to 60 seconds between each of the three sets. The sprinting should be followed by stretching exercises.

    d. *Flexibility Exercises.* Continue using stretch exercise 1, 3, 7, and 10 in GAF Level II program, and add 2, 6, 8, and 9 (pages 100, 108, 112, 114).

Note: Most ballplayers forget about flexibility once the game begins despite the evidence that most of their time is spent standing and sitting in the dugout. Although most players warm up their arms when they come out of the dugout, they ignore their legs. Get the habit of doing a few hamstring and groin stretches before returning to the defensive position and before stepping into the batter's box.

1. Players, other than the pitcher and catcher, who weigh 117 pounds will burn about 220 calories per hour; the 150-pound person will burn about 280 calories.

2. Baseball and softball are moderate-activity sports.

3. Baseball should be limited to the under-40 age-group as a weekend activity. The slower reaction of those over the age of 40 involves a real risk of being hit by the ball.

Softball may be played at any age if all the players are approximately of the same age and ability. However, the custom of putting the oldest and slowest person on the pitcher's mound in slow-pitch softball should be stopped. The pitcher should always be able to react quickly to avoid being hit by a sharply rapped ball.

4. Both games require good muscular strength of the arms, shoulder girdle, and grip. Legs require good strength and endurance. Flexibility of the shoulders, lower back, and hamstring muscles is essential.

5. A high level of cardiorespiratory fitness is unnecessary but is certainly helpful. However, anaerobic conditioning is important because sprints of 50 yards or less are common.

Basketball Basketball is now played by the Chinese and Czechs, the Saudis and Soviets, in Africa and the Arctic, in most nations of the world. Hoops are screwed to the sides of houses and barns, to poles and palm trees. Basketball is easy to learn, never dull, so challenging that many of us find it impossible to give up. We met weekenders age 40 and over who run three nights a week only because they need the conditioning to play basketball on three other nights. At West Point the annual Over-35 Basketball Tournament includes one participant who has passed age 60.

Basketball is played by old and young men and by children, and if kids don't have a hoop, they nail a peach basket to a wall just as James Naismith did—and we would like to stand still for a half dozen sentences to pay homage to Naismith, the Canadian who invented basketball. Naismith was an instructor at the International Young Men's Christian Association, Springfield, Massachusetts, in

1891, when the department head asked him to think of something to relieve the boredom of calisthenics between the football and baseball seasons.

Naismith cut the bottoms out of two peach baskets and nailed them to the balcony 10 feet above the floor at either end of the gymnasium. The rules he developed—including no running with the ball, anyone can shoot, both teams can occupy the same area, no personal contact, only the hands can be used—are still basic to the game. Within a year basketball was being played at eastern colleges and as far west as the University of Iowa. At Cornell, in 1892, basketball was played with 50 men on a side—100 men on the floor!

Basketball is more than a game because it has had an enormous impact on physical fitness. A vigorous activity, its popularity has required that millions of participants show up in reasonably good physical condition.

BODY PARTS

Basketball is strenuous when played competitively and demands excellent physical fitness. If legs, ankles, and feet are not properly conditioned, the lower body suffers ankle sprains and strains, muscle pulls of the hamstrings and groin, Achilles tendinitis, quadriceps contusions, and knee injuries. Strong hands, arms, and shoulders are necessary to handle the ball in a crowd.

For the weekend or occasional player, the most important parts are the muscles of the lower body and the cardiorespiratory system. Proper conditioning should include strength-building and flexibility exercises.

CONDITIONING

1. General Athletic Fitness. The GAF Level III conditioning program is required to meet the heavy-activity rating of basketball. The extra cardiorespiratory conditioning in the Extra Edge is absolutely necessary if you wish to be able to play your best and enjoy the game.

2. Specific Athletic Fitness. Prior to the basketball season you should be able to perform at GAF Level III without undue fatigue. During the season continue with the GAF Level III workout two or three times a week. On alternate days work at the CR condi-

tioning in Extra Edge plus some rope jumping and stretching exercises. In addition to the GAF flexibility exercises 1, 5, 8, and 9 (pages 98, 106, 112, 114), stretch out with Flexibility Exercises 2, 4, 6, and 7 (pages 100, 104, 108, 110). Use the same flexibility exercises for warm-up and cool-down periods.

Additional SAF calisthenics on alternate days should include:

a. High Jumper (see GAF Level III, page 169).

b. Kangaroo Hop (see SAF for Downhill Skiing, page 301).

HEALTH AND FITNESS ANALYSIS

1. A 117-pound person playing the usually vigorous weekend game will burn about 400 calories per hour; a 150-pound person, 525 calories.

2. Basketball rates as a heavy-activity sport and requires sound SAF and GAF conditioning to play your best and avoid injury.

3. Basketball can be played by well-conditioned athletes at almost any age. Realistically, however, few continue to play after their forties. Former college and high school players who "come out of retirement" should take it easy. Begin slowly with some shooting, passing, and dribbling after each conditioning workout. It takes time before the old skills return. As a general rule, players in their forties and over should play against opponents of about the same age.

West Point's Over-35 Basketball Tournament comes close to equalizing abilities for the mature set. It is a well-organized tournament with set teams, officiated games, and trophies for the winning team. By contrast, when the Noontime Pickup Basketball League meets during the lunch hour, the first five players to appear form one team; the next five, the opponents. As additional players arrive, they organize a third team and wait for one of the first two teams to score ten baskets. The team must also be at least two baskets ahead to be declared the winner.

The winning team remains on the floor and plays the next team. This continues as long as ten players are available. Fouls are called by the person who is fouled, but no free throws are allowed. The fouled team takes the ball at the "top of the key" and puts it into play.

4. Strength and flexibility of the lower body are essential to play well and avoid injuries to the lower body. Upper-body strength will

improve your game but is not critical in preventing injuries.

5. Unless you play only "horse," * cardiorespiratory fitness is an absolute prerequisite for basketball. You get in shape to play basketball rather than play basketball to get in shape. In fact, conditioning is often more important than skill in weekend games. Skilled players may start with a bang, but as fatigue sets in, the well-conditioned team will catch up and win.

Soccer   Soccer is the world's most popular sport, number one in seventy different countries. Major matches draw up to 150,000 spectators, far more than the Super Bowl. Soccer is an Olympic event, but the most prestigious competition is reserved for the World Cup Matches, which occur every four years. In Great Britain soccer is called association football, and in most other countries simply "football." Soccer has come lately to the United States, but in recent years its popularity has been booming and for good reason.

Soccer has some of the characteristics and excitement of basketball. It is a continuous game, easy to learn, the ball moves all over the playing area, and everyone plays the ball. Unlike American football, the ball is always out in the open, and there are no set plays. The game develops individual initiative and ability.

Soccer was first played in the United States in 1869 in a regulation game between Princeton and Rutgers. Today soccer has spread down to elementary schools. It may be the best developmental sport for children because more than any other game it requires both mental and physical agility.

BODY PARTS

Soccer requires excellent conditioning of the lower body and the cardiorespiratory systems because the sport demands a lot of running. The arms and shoulders are important for the throw-in but take lesser conditioning.

The most common injuries occur to the ankles (sprains and broken bones), feet (broken bones), leg cramps, and shin splints.

---

* A shooting game that requires virtually no action. The lead player chooses to make any shot. If the leader or any other player misses the same shot, the player gets a letter from the word H-O-R-S-E. The leader then makes a different shot and the competition continues. The player who has five misses accumulates all the letters, HORSE, and is eliminated from the competition.

However, good physical conditioning will largely prevent these injuries.

CONDITIONING

1. General Athletic Fitness. As a heavy-activity sport, soccer requires a conditioning program at GAF Level III. Plenty of running is also necessary, so be certain to do the GAF Extra Edge cardiorespiratory program. Aerobic conditioning is more important than anaerobic because the game requires continuous running. However, wind spirits improve performance and are therefore included in SAF.

2. Specific Athletic Fitness. For the weekend soccer player who is not engaged in daily, specific practice sessions, the GAF Level III workout should be scheduled at least three times a week. On alternate days, specific activities must be practiced to develop skills and athletic fitness. Rope jumping is both a good agility and cardiorespiratory conditioning activity. Other specific exercises include:

a. *Sprints.* These are necessary as a complement, not as a supplement, to the Extra Edge program. See instructions for sprinting under "Baseball/Softball" on page 337. For soccer, first do the sprints without the ball; then add the ball, and sprint the same distances while dribbling.

b. *Flexibility Exercises.* Continue with the GAF Level III flexibility exercises 1, 5, 8, and 9 and add 2, 3, 6, and 7 (see pages 100, 102, 108, 110).

c. *Hand Kick* (see page 343).

HAND KICK

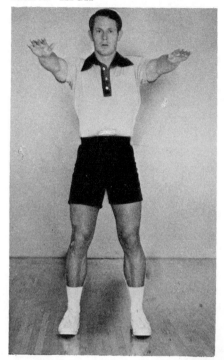

STARTING
POSITION

COUNT 1

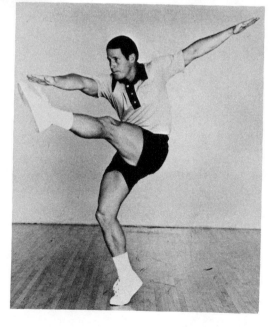

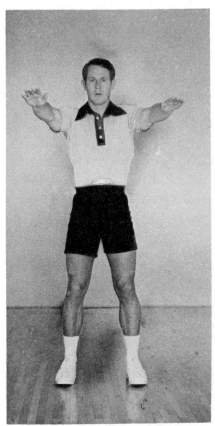

COUNT 2

COUNT 3

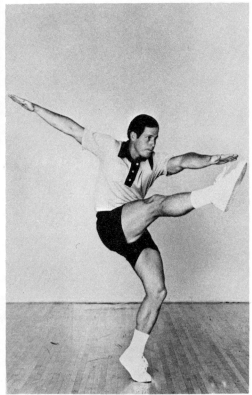

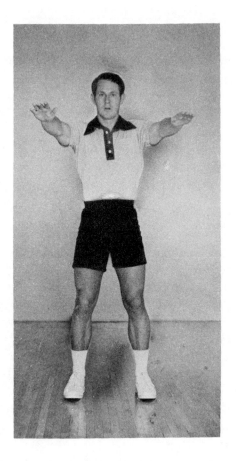

COUNT 4

Starting Position: Stand with feet separated to shoulder width, arms extended to the front, parallel to each other and horizontal to the ground.

Action: Count 1: Using the left leg, try to kick the right hand, and return to the starting position.

Count 2: Using the right leg, try to kick the left hand, and return to starting position.

Count 3: Repeat Count 1.

Count 4: Repeat Count 2.

Cadence: Moderate to fast.

Progression: Begin with 10 repetitions, and gradually increase to 20 repetitions.

Other specific exercises are found in soccer drills, which include passing, kicking, and throwing the ball in from out of bounds. Use the flexibility exercises before and after practice.

Cardiorespiratory exercises through running, rope jumping, and sprinting must be emphasized. A Russian study of 110 soccer matches and 200 training sessions by Vojin N. Smodlaka, M.D., Sc.D., found that in 90 minutes of the game a player spends 30 to 32 minutes running, 50 to 58 minutes walking, and only 53 to 60 seconds standing. The importance of sprinting is underlined by a count of 48 to 78 starts in place, 40 to 62 accelerations, and 1 to 15 jumps. In addition, there were 14 to 42 fights for the ball.

HEALTH AND FITNESS ANALYSIS

1. A 117-pound person playing a typical weekend soccer game uses about 415 calories per hour; a 150-pound person, 540 calories.

2. Soccer is a heavy-activity sport that requires excellent GAF and SAF conditioning to compete and avoid injury.

3. Soccer can be enjoyed by both sexes and for many years, but weekenders in their mid-forties should beg off playing with youngsters. Unlike limited-area sports, such as squash, handball, racquetball, and tennis, where skills and experience count, soccer is played on fields that are as long as or longer than football fields, where physical superiority is the advantage.

Soccer should preferably be learned in the preteens or teens, played in the twenties and thirties if you are in good condition, and then taught in the forties.

Parents should note that soccer may be the best of game-learning experiences for young children and is especially superior to American football for prepubescent youngsters. Soccer does a better job of teaching body balance and agility than football. A youngster can learn to punt, kick, run, throw, and catch without pads. Furthermore, the incidence of injury among children is virtually nil. Of course, children, like adults, should also have the advantage and preparation of preconditioning.

4. Muscular strength and flexibility of both legs are extremely important. The trunk muscles should also be strong and flexible.

5. In a regulation game of two forty-five-minute periods, a soccer player may run as many as 8 to 10 miles, underlining the importance of cardiorespiratory conditioning. In fact, the better-condi-

tioned team usually wins over the better-skilled, poorly conditioned team. Joe Palone's secret as West Point's soccer coach for twenty-five years was fielding the best-conditioned team. He was recognized as one of the most successful coaches in college soccer, although he seldom had the most skilled players.

Touch/Flag Football   Touch or flag football ranks as one of the weekend athlete's most popular pickup games. And that explains why there are so many injuries after the Saturday or Sunday afternoon game. We underestimate the demands of the sport because it is so easy to get a game going. Touch football can be played anywhere—on the street, a vacant lot, the beach, or the deck of a ship. All you need is a ball and people.

There are no universally recognized standardized rules for touch football, so the kinds and amount of contact will vary. The ball-carrier is stopped either by a one-hand or two-hand tag or by an opponent's grabbing one of the flags that is tucked in the belt on each side. Sometimes blocking is permitted, but blockers cannot leave their feet or use their hands.

Many weekenders innocently believe that touch football is a light game because rough body contact is eliminated. In fact, touch football is a very vigorous game. Many of the "little, light injuries" result in leg casts and weeks of rehabilitation.

BODY PARTS

Touch football is a total body activity. Although passing requires strong, flexible arms and shoulders, the running, dodging, and cutting make lower-body conditioning more important. Predictably most injuries, including sprained ankles and knees, are to the lower limbs. Occasionally hands are injured in catching or tagging. Some of this may be prevented by the removal of rings and other jewelry. Finally, because of the intensive running and sprinting, aerobic and anaerobic conditioning is necessary.

CONDITIONING

1. General Athletic Fitness. The running, blocking, passing, catching, and tagging make touch football a heavy-activity sport. For the competitive player, GAF Level III conditioning is absolutely necessary. Unfortunately, if injury is to be avoided, the same level of

conditioning is necessary for the person who plays only once a year at the company picnic.

2. Specific Athletic Fitness. Specific conditioning for all touch football players includes:

a. Cardiorespiratory conditioning in addition to that in GAF Level III. Use the Extra Edge program, and complement this with an anaerobic workout, sprinting (page 337).

b. Flexibility exercises 2, 3, 6, and 7 (pages 100, 102, 108, 110), in addition to 1, 5, 8, and 9 under GAF Level III. Use these for preconditioning and for warm-up and cool-down periods.

Some exercises are specific to the position you play. A quarterback must get his arm in shape. If for only one game, begin throwing the ball at least two weeks before the event. Start by throwing short passes, and gradually work up to your normal range. Do not try to throw 65 yards when 40 yards is your best distance. We know of weekenders who "come out of retirement" at age 30 and try to pass farther than they did at age 25. Not likely unless you have been into some long-term arm strengthening.

If you are the punter or kickoff man, spend two or three weeks prior to the game working with the Hand Kick (page 343).

HEALTH AND FITNESS ANALYSIS

1. A 117-pound person playing a typically vigorous game of weekend touch football will use about 300 calories per hour; a 150-pound person, 390 calories.

2. Touch/flag football is a heavy-activity sport that requires a lot of running, usually over relatively short distances of 50 yards or less, and some contact. Because of the pickup nature of the game, many players are not properly conditioned, and injuries to the lower limbs are common.

3. Touch/flag football should be learned in the preteens and teens, played in the twenties and thirties if participants are properly conditioned, and viewed as a spectator in the forties.

4. Muscular strength and flexibility of the legs and trunk are very important. For passers and catchers, the strength and flexibility of the shoulders are also important.

5. Cardiorespiratory fitness should be both aerobic, using the GAF Level III Extra Edge running program, and anaerobic, using the sprinting program. Just as in regular football, injuries usually

are more prevalent after the half time break, because of inadequate warm-ups before the second half, and during the fourth quarter, when fatigue becomes a factor.

Volleyball In the 1890's Holyoke, Massachusetts businessmen didn't like the way the basketball was bouncing at the local YMCA. The newly invented (1891), newfangled basketball game was too strenuous for them. In 1895 the Y's physical director, William G. Morgan, invented volleyball for older members. However, the younger generation muscled in, and volleyball's popularity gradually spread throughout the states and across the oceans. Before volleyball was accepted by the International Olympics Committee in 1957, world championship matches were held in Prague, Paris, and Moscow.

Today volleyball is played competitively in high schools and colleges. At a highly competitive level volleyball is a vigorous and exciting sport. The word's best teams come from Asia and eastern Europe. Americans are gradually beginning to improve, but we are still a few years away from competing on an even basis with the men's teams from Russia and Poland, and what some of these teams do with a volleyball is amazing. However, the game can also be enjoyed at a recreational level or on the sandlot.

BODY PARTS

The body must be well conditioned for high-level volleyball. The game demands jumping ability, speed of movement, and excellent hand-eye coordination. Playground volleyball requires good leg strength and good flexibility of the arms, shoulders, and legs. The offensive and defensive patterns in highly competitive volleyball are intricate, but on the playground the game is simple and great fun.

The injuries in volleyball are normally the same regardless of the ability of the players. Ankle sprains and fractures, shin splints, and knee injuries occur because of the jumping. Shoulder injuries and sprained wrists and fingers come from blocking spikes or from spiking the ball incorrectly.

CONDITIONING

1. General Athletic Fitness. Top-level volleyball rates as a heavy-activity sport, but few weekend athletes play at that level. There-

fore, volleyball rates as a moderate activity with GAF Level II conditioning appropriate for most weekend athletes. However, for those playing in a highly competitive league, GAF Level III conditioning is recommended.

2. Specific Athletic Fitness. Specific movements such as setting, jumping, spiking, serving, and diving require extra-good body flexibility. All ten of the GAF flexibility exercises (pages 98–117) should be part of your SAF conditioning program.

SAF exercises to strengthen your legs are:

a. *Step-ups* (see page 166).

b. *High Jumper* (see page 169).

Additional practice drills should be scheduled to develop timing for the specific activities of serving, setting, and spiking.

3. Preactivity Warm-up/Postgame Cool-off. Do all of the ten flexibility exercises, and then practice specific serving, setting and spiking drills.

HEALTH AND FITNESS ANALYSIS

1. A 117-pound person playing the typical weekend game of volleyball will burn 270 calories per hour; in a highly competitive game, 460 calories. The 150-pound person will burn 350 calories per hour; 600 calories in high-level competition.

2. For the normal weekend player, volleyball is a moderate-activity sport; for the highly competitive participant, a heavy-activity sport. Good conditioning is important at both levels of activity to prevent injuries and guarantee good performance.

3. Volleyball may be played by virtually all age-groups. The level of play is dependent on the level of conditioning. The chance of injuries increases when age-groups are mixed. Eventually a younger person will spike a ball hard at an older opponent whose reflexes may not be equal to the action, and the older person may be hurt. As with most sports, volleyball is most enjoyable when teams are evenly matched.

4. Muscular strength and flexibility of the legs and shoulders are very important for all volleyball players.

5. Volleyball itself does little to develop cardiorespiratory fitness because of the stop-and-start nature of the game. However, cardiorespiratory fitness is essential to maintain vigor in volleyball. Follow the Extra Edge running program at the appropriate GAF level.

Rope skipping should be considered an important adjunct to your conditioning program.

Grip Strength

Grip strength is probably the most neglected factor among weekend athletes. Perhaps that is understandable. We use our hands continuously during our waking hours and assume that our grip is the least of our conditioning problems. It is a common mistake. We learned that at West Point when women entered the Academy. Most had difficulty handling a 10-pound rifle.

We knew that the women's upper-torso strength was far below that of the men because few of the women cadets could do pull-ups. At first we thought that was the only problem. When we came to realize that the lack of grip strength was a major factor, we put them on a simple grip-strengthening program. Their performance in handling military equipment improved, and so did their performance on the courts and field when handling balls and racquets.

Happily, grip-strength exercises are simple and easy and take little time. They can be worked any time without warm-up or cool-down exercises while you are reading or talking on the telephone, but remember to give both hands a workout.

BALL SQUEEZE

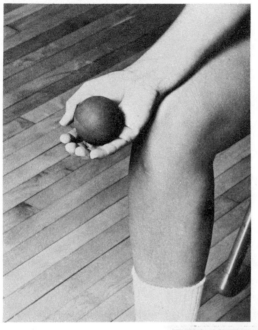

STARTING POSITION

COUNT 1

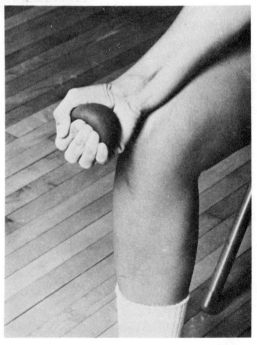

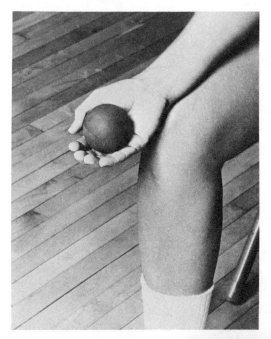

COUNT 2

COUNT 3

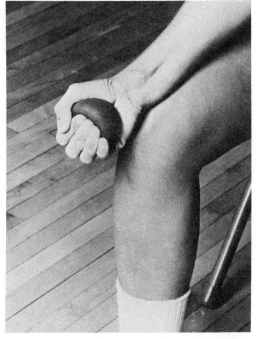

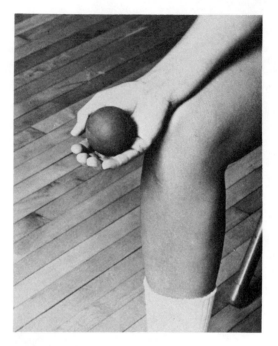

COUNT 4

Ball Squeeze

Equipment: A sponge rubber ball slightly smaller than a tennis ball; a racquetball is the ideal size. Or use one of the grip-strength developers (see illustration).

Starting Position: While standing, sitting, or walking, hold the ball or implement in the palm of your hand.

Action: Count 1: Slowly squeeze the ball, taking about 2 or 3 seconds to complete the contraction, and then hold the contraction for a count of 3 seconds.

   Count 2: Release the grip for 1 second.

   Count 3: Repeat Count 1.

   Count 4: Release the grip for 1 second.

Cadence: Slow.

TOWEL TWIST

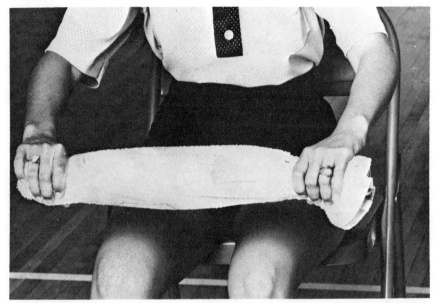

STARTING POSITION

COUNT 1

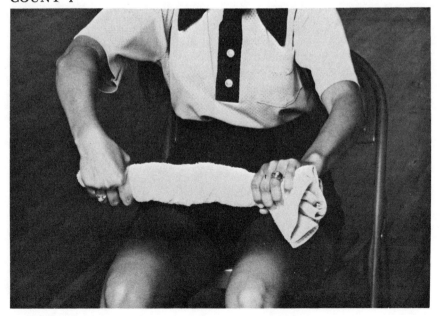

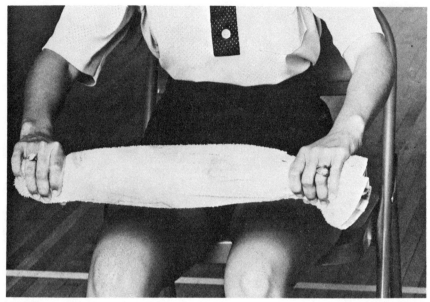

COUNT 2

COUNT 3

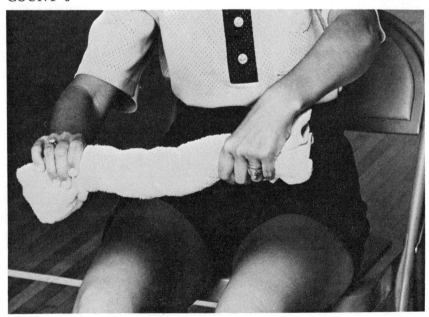

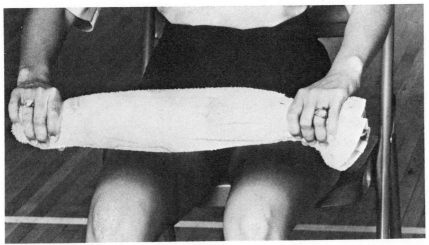

COUNT 4

Towel Twist

Equipment: One small towel.

Starting Position: Roll the towel lengthwise until it is about 2 to 3 inches in diameter. Hold the towel at both ends with palms facing down.

Action: Count 1: Twist the towel, and continue twisting until it is in a hard knot.

Count 2: Relax and shake the knot out of the towel.

Count 3: Repeat Count 1, twisting the towel in the opposite direction.

Count 4: Repeat Count 2.

Exercise Notes

1. Continue the above exercises until the muscles of the hands and forearms are completely fatigued.

2. Do not use these exercises before a game, but work out with them afterward.

3. For faster results, work with these exercises once a day and every day.

4. Do not use these exercises if you have hypertension. Both exercises will raise your blood pressure.

PART V

The Psychological Edge

Getting Up/Staying Up

Chapter 21

The Psychological Edge

Most of this book has been concerned with physical preparation —and it goes without saying that if you go into a game when you're out of condition, it's the equivalent of playing with blisters and a stretched waistband. There you are, hurting and trying to hold up your shorts and, at the same time, trying to maintain concentration and confidence. It won't work. If you're out of shape, you're out of the running. On the other hand, it would be very wrong to underestimate the importance of psychological conditioning.

The study of sports psychology is a twentieth-century science. The Russians pioneered, as early as 1917, when their laboratories began to examine the special psychology of athletes. Today Russian sports technologists test children at the age of 9 or younger for their sports aptitude. If a kid kicks a ball pretty well but is too individualistic, he may be directed away from a team sport such as soccer. A youngster with too much self-esteem had better think of boxing, running, or swimming, activities that require no team play. The Russians pair personality with a specific sport, and if the child athlete does not score well in both, the youngster becomes a reject at age 10.

Generally the Russians come from the school of behavioral psychology that relies on the carrot and stick for motivation. Rewards and gratification keep the youngster in line. The child gets better food, better clothes, and pocket money as long as progress is made. If not, the child loses the whole bag and gets thrown back into the communal pond.

By contrast, American sports during most of this century have been a mom-and-pop operation. Our top athletes have been nurtured in the home and sandlots. Often parents make a great sacrifice with enormous expenditures of energy, effort, and the family's savings to acquire professional coaching during a youngster's early years. We have found this acceptable. As a people we honor individualism and self-initiative.

In addition, we tolerate an individual's self-esteem in team sports. As a result, many of our greatest hitters, pitchers, and other athletes appear to be among the most conceited persons in the country, although in truth so are many of our superstars in science, business, the arts, and politics. Again, as a people we have learned to accept personality differences, and furthermore, the prima donnas often carry a team to a division or world title.

Because American psychologists are also concerned with the preservation of individualism and initiative, they focus on individual traits that strengthen the person as well as the separate psychological problems, such as concentration and mental preparation, that specifically affect performance.

In 1922 Coleman Griffin, of the University of Illinois, published *Psychology of Athletes*, the first American study of sports psychology. His book was virtually ignored by coaches. It was not until the late 1950's and early 1960's that American psychologists again took sports into the laboratories. Today the rhetoric of psychology pervades sports pages and locker rooms, but much of it has become a meaningless cacophony of buzz words. We would like to get away from some of the nonsense and misunderstandings. Furthermore, we will interpret the research for its practical application because most of the studies in sports psychology are complicated and abstract.

In the first part of this book, we separated physiological matter into general and specific conditioning, and there's a similar parallel in sports psychology. The technology of psychology is rooted in subjective attitudes toward sports. Even the prima donnas of the sports world subscribe to the Western world's concept of fair play and sportsmanship. When we talked to a weekend athlete who was psychologically inept, we found that part of the problem lay in his misunderstanding of why people participate in sports.

We met Nick, a weekend athlete in his late thirties, who has always been a good athlete. Off the courts he's mannered and responsible, but in a game he makes a poor partner or opponent. His need to score edges on the desperate. When he is losing, he rages within himself. He self-destructs. His whole athletic experience thus becomes unsatisfactory. There's no chance of his coming into a game with the right mental preparation because he lacks the right feeling for competition, and that's ironic and sad. Where did he get the idea that winning is the only thing? From his parents? His high school or college coach? Or Vince Lombardi?

Lombardi said: "Winning isn't everything. It's the only thing."

Lombardi's statement has had an overwhelming impact on the spirit of competition and psychological principles of competition. The Lombardi maxim has been adopted by corporate executives, at least one President of the United States, and too many athletes. All have failed to understand what he was saying.

West Point's famed Football Coach Red Blaik knew Lombardi intimately. They were friends who golfed together and professional colleagues who spent thousands of hours together discussing football strategy. Blaik believes that Lombardi was paraphrasing Gen. Douglas MacArthur's statement "There is no substitute for victory." But MacArthur was talking about war. War is a life-or-death situation. All the prospects of defeat are grim. Although West Point officers are highly competitive weekend athletes, often to the great annoyance of their spouses when playing mixed doubles, West Pointers understand the differences between war and sports. And so did Vince Lombardi. Lombardi never intended to say that a sports loss entailed the death of the spirit.

Cadets who knew Lombardi when he coached at West Point always understood he was saying that striving to win is everything, that striving is the only thing. In researching this book, we questioned Red Blaik, whom Lombardi identified as his mentor.

Blaik noted, "I don't pretend to speak for Lombardi, but the idea that winning justifies the means was totally unacceptable to him and any other sane coach. What he was saying, and what we believed, is that to accept defeat without rebelling within yourself is shameful as you will accept the next defeat with less concern and eventually say to yourself, 'What the hell.' Thus, stalemate becomes acceptable and even desirable."

Every successful competitor, no matter what the endeavor, understands what Blaik is saying: If man hadn't rebelled against adversity, we would still be back in the Stone Age, and no matter what you may think about the present world, it's a lot better. In fact, attitudes toward sports activity are a lot better today than they were only a couple of thousand years ago.

Dartmouth professor and novelist Erich Segal, an ardent weekend athlete, reminds us: "The single aim in Greek athletics was to win. There were no awards for second place; in fact, losing was considered a disgrace."

Today Penn State's outstanding Football Coach Joe Paterno reminds us that when competitors strive to win, "There's enough glory in the game for everybody—winners and losers."

The key is the will to strive.

We are talking about this because the weekend athlete is the most important athlete in the world not only in number but in the context of the competitive spirit. The weekender is not concerned with winning a better contract or international prestige. The weekender has the rare opportunity to experience the unique unity of mind and body, free of material rewards.

In what follows we are using an alphabetical format similar to a concise encyclopedia. Some of the entries, such as "Fair Play" and "Sportsmanship," are subjective because we would like you to come to terms with the true meanings of these timeworn words. Other entries, such as "Game Plan" and "Mental Preparation," go to the specifics of winning. You may go directly to one or the other with the understanding that all the entries are independent.

Aggression   Is aggressive behavior something worth developing? What are the implications of aggression? These questions bewilder many head coaches. They walk around complaining that a particular athlete is not aggressive and worry about what they can do about it.

Are these coaches thinking straight?

Are the glaring and growling of bulldog behavior something to be desired?

What does aggressive behavior mean to the weekend athlete?

If you get a survival twinge when you're up against an aggressive opponent, your gut feeling is valid. You should be apprehensive. To the sports psychologist, aggression has at its base the intent to cause injury. That is not good, and that is not what most coaches want.

Competitive? Yes.

Enterprising? Yes.

Tough? Yes.

But don't confuse aggressive behavior with either drive or initiative.

When facing an aggressive opponent, take the counsel of a highly competitive essayist that one "Rides the whirlwind and directs the storm."

Anger   There's no place for hostility in sports competition. Stop the game, and talk it out. If your opponent turns out to be "naturally obnoxious," find someone else to play with.

Anxiety   There is a specific type of anxiety known to actors, athletes, astronauts, and others before lift-off called the butterflies. The flutters occur in the stomach and may range in intensity from a queasy feeling to nausea.

Because you are uncertain of the outcome, pregame anxiety is natural, even helpful. It is a positive sign that the body is gearing up for a challenge. Therefore, you will be playing harder, lifting your performance, to ensure that the outcome is pleasurable. And the more important the contest, the more likely the anxiety.

Once a performance begins, the anxiety disappears and is replaced by concentration and intent. If you suffer from anxiety throughout a game, see "Mental Preparation," "Game Plan," and "Concentration."

Aptitude   Is there an athletic aptitude? Should you worry about your ability and capacity for a specific sport? Can you switch sports, add sports with ease?

Part II lists the general qualities of performance and explains that most can be improved with conditioning and practice. You can also assess your qualifications for specific sports. For instance, if you are fairly quick at one racquet sport, you can play most other racquet sports. The reason: The smaller the playing area, the quicker you have to be.

If you are thinking of adding or switching sports, turn to "SAF—Specific Athletic Conditioning" (page 241). Compare the body parts used in the sport that you are now playing with the one that you are contemplating. This will help you analyze how well you can do and how to prepare for the new game. If both sports require similar use of the body, you should be able to learn the new game in short order.

A weekend athlete would be foolish to worry about mental aptitude. If you have too much self-esteem, turn it into motivation to improve your physical condition. If you're a high achiever, seek out tough competitors. If you have a problem with your temper, see "Aggression," "Fair Play," "Frustration," and "Sportsmanship."

The degree of aptitude is important only to psychologists and the coach who is developing a champion or championship team. Most of us play for fun. A few weekend athletes will become trophy winners, but neither aptitude nor trophies should be the weekender's criteria for trying out a new sport. Give it a chance. Give yourself a chance. If the activity is gratifying, compete at your best level. Don't worry about aptitude.

Arousal (Pumping Up/Juicing Up) After the Steelers' victory at Super Bowl XIV Terry Bradshaw said, "I think I played more of a leadership role in this game. I was talking pretty good in the huddle. They knew I wanted this one bad. I juiced them."

Arousal is the reason behind locker-room pep talks and quarterback juicing. The home-field advantage is basically the excitement generated by the support of hometown fans at the game and rallies. Even sports reporters stir up arousal with player-by-player interviews before a big game.

It should be noted that arousal may also be stirred by challenges that are almost entirely internal. In 1954, when Roger Bannister broke the four-minute mile, the story made front-page headlines around the world. Everyone had thought that the feat was impossible. The arousal was self-generated.

When Sir Roger, now a physician, talks about his feelings before the run, he recalls, "The four-minute mile had become rather like an Everest, a challenge to the human spirit. It was a barrier that seemed to defy all attempts to break it—an irksome reminder that man's striving might be in vain."

Arousal is a vital factor in gaining a competitive edge. An excited state prepares the physiological and psychological organism for action. It lifts your game and sometimes results in superb performance. However, arousal must be managed.

Since the Yerkes-Dodson Law was formulated, we have learned that pre-event arousal must be contained to improve performance. Beyond certain arousal levels, performance drops; tension sets in and interferes with performance. This is called the inverted-U relationship.

YERKES-DODSON LAW

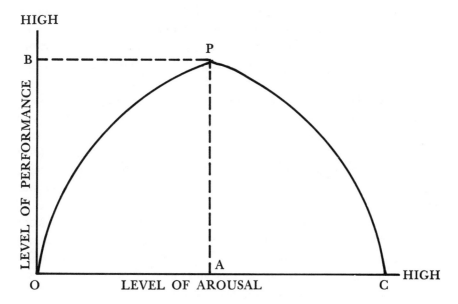

As the arousal level increases from zero to point A, the level of performance increases as described by the curve from zero to point P. However, as the level of arousal continues to go higher, the level of performance will drop as described by the curve from P to C.

The weekend athlete has no trouble getting up for a game when playing someone who is better than he. In most instances, the weekender should welcome pregame excitement and help create arousal especially if the game is routine. Friendly rivals indulge in pregame kidding or make small wagers (see "Betting, Friendly"). All this has to be done with a measure of awareness and control to forestall escalation of tension. We have to be especially careful of being overcharged when playing in a tournament or before friends and family. And we have to avoid being intimidated internally when we have a chance at grabbing a big win. Pitcher Tom Seaver recalls that when he discovered that he was going for a no-hitter, he cooled it by telling himself, "If it happens, it happens." Other keys to preventing overarousal are in the entries "Concentration," "Game Plan," and "Mental Preparation."

Associate/Disassociate　The mind acts in mysterious ways. Many of us have blocked out pain during a highly contested game to discover later that we required the services of a physician. Studies of pain during combat find that some soldiers can escape the agony of a wound by manipulating their thoughts. This is disassociation, the body's way of coping with trauma. Unfortunately a number of athletes have learned to use disassociation routinely.

Some weekend marathoners don't want to face up to the long miles ahead of them and don't want to pay the price of aches and discomfort that come with the territory. Instead, they play mental games with themselves to shut out reality. They go on highs, a kind of self-hypnosis that sends their minds far away to a pleasant situation, perhaps to bask on a sunny beach. They successfully block out sensory feedback. It is very risky.

Marathon runner Bill Rodgers and other elite athletes in other sports will tell you that they never have highs, never disassociate while competing. Instead, they learn to monitor and use body signals to improve their performances and prevent injuries. This is a practice that every weekender, whatever the sport activity, should learn. It may result in helping you pace yourself in order to maintain momentum. At the least it will keep a simple injury from being aggravated. Part III, "Body Parts: Their Care and Maintenance," should help you learn to interpret sensory feedback. Also, see the entry "Paying the Price" in this section.

Break the habit of disassociating. Your body is one of your best friends. Keep in touch.

Betting, Friendly　Betting on sports is occasionally illegal and always popular. When betting more than you can afford to lose, you had better be a cool cat in order to avoid excessive tension. On the other hand, betting a beer or soda often adds a reasonable degree of arousal. It serves to remind friendly opponents, the best kind, that no matter how often you play against one another, you are playing to win.

Challenge In discussing competition from foreign-made automobiles, Thomas A. Murphy, chairman of General Motors, said, "We've risen to every challenge, and we're going to be tougher than ever."

Accepting or seeking out challenge is as important in performance and winning as conditioning and technique are. In accepting a challenge, you implicitly agree to test your mental and physical resources. You raise the arousal level; that explains why the underdog doesn't need to bet on himself. In any field of endeavor, from business to sports, it's challenge that provides the exhilaration.

One weekend athlete, James Ford, chaplain of the U.S. House of Representatives, constantly looks for challenges above and beyond saving sinners. His sports interests have ranged from the courts to hot-dogging on ski slopes. In his lifetime he has biked up and down mountains, skied backward off a ski jump, shot white waters, and sailed the width of the Atlantic Ocean in a 31-foot craft.

When Jim Ford talks about challenge, he may recall one special incident to define his feelings, a winter morning on a mountaintop in New Hampshire with a skiing companion. Just as they were to push off on the run down the mountainside, Ford recalls that their exhilaration was raised to exultation, and the two men sang the doxology.

We don't know whether the best and brightest seek out challenge or whether challenge itself brightens the best, the way a bright child presented with a new puzzle or game may complain that it's "too easy." However, we do know that challenge hones the competitive edge and makes the blood sing.

Choking Most golfers experience choking while standing over a three-foot putt on the final hole to determine who wins the match. The golfer may look calm when, in fact, excessive tension is present in the muscles. This is an excellent illustration of the Yerkes-Dodson Law (see "Arousal").

Choking can be overcome by experience and mental preparation. In the brief time that you take to line up the shot, allow yourself an instant to remember how pleasurable it felt the last time you succeeded in making a similar putt. Recalling the pleasure may help relax your muscles long enough to repeat the success.

If your memory bank is blank, take a deep breath and yawn. Or sneeze. Or when you are cagily squinting at the turf, allow yourself two seconds to relax, and imagine the long, cool drink waiting for you at the clubhouse and swallow slowly. Anything that relaxes your muscles may help win the game.

Class   John Kelley has twice won the Boston Marathon. At age 71, when he finished his forty-eighth Boston Marathon, he said, "I got tired the last couple of miles, but I never stopped running."

Code   President John G. Kemeny, Dartmouth College, counselling a new freshman class: "Don't compromise; don't make excuses."

Commitment   Go back to an old cliché: If something is worth doing, it's worth doing well. To be a good weekend athlete, you must be involved. You must develop the unity of mind and body. There is no other way.

Competition   Not a dirty word. Not, as some critics contend, the poison in our society, but as Shimon Peres, Israeli political leader, observes, "Wherever you have freedom, you have competition." Without competition, there is no opportunity, no choice. The spirit withers. Furthermore, we are discovering that sports competition in itself, when encouraged, improves the quality of life. A study of male and female industrial workers found that active participation in competitive sports was correlated with better interpersonal relations as well as more interest and satisfaction in their work.

At West Point all cadets are required to compete in athletics, including those who did not compete before coming to the Academy. We know that sports competition offers great opportunities to develop the unified personality and to learn to lead and follow. Athletes learn to give and take. Team members must commit themselves to the good of the common cause. Through competitive athletics one learns to win and lose and to accept the consequences of her or his own actions.

The cadets learn that there is exhilaration in responsibility, a lesson well known to all athletes. Former pitcher Sandy Koufax once said, "When you're playing, you think, 'Why did it have to come down to me again?' But once you're away from baseball you see how much you enjoyed the responsibility."

None of these comments is the exclusive insight of athletes. Some years ago, a California lawyer gave this advice to a son who was entering West Point:

"Look, son. This is no junior country club you are going to. You will compete for everything, but with men who will be your best friends for life. Don't ever quit."

Concentration All of us have had times when we played well one day and dismally the next. It doesn't make sense because you can't lose skills or get out of condition in twenty-four hours. The nemesis, the monster of competition, is the failure of concentration. It is insidious because we often don't realize it is happening, and it happens to all of us.

When Tony Dorsett reported to the Dallas Cowboys, he noted that he hadn't fully developed all his talents and that he especially had to work on his concentration—a wise assessment, acknowledging that concentration can be learned and developed.

By definition, concentration is the focusing of skills on a goal-oriented task. It is an abstract concept, and redundant, what with concentration, focus, and goal-oriented being closely related words. Despite this, we can identify several elements involved in concentration.

One factor in maintaining concentration is control of the environment. At one level this is relatively easy and depends on physical isolation. A student closes the bedroom door and takes the phone off the hook to prepare for an oral examination. A business executive tells a secretary to hold all calls in order to consolidate notes for a policy paper. What weekend athletes fail to understand is that sports competition requires similar preparation.

A pro football player, whose name escapes us, is known to walk around the stadium several times before entering the locker room to dress for the game. A sportswriter interpreted this as a kind of superstition. In fact, the athlete was warming up his concentration. Sue Tendy, coach of the women's swimming team at West Point, also competes at the masters' level in international swimming events. Before competition, she gets off by herself for thirty minutes. What is happening here is that the athlete is closing the door on personal matters and the other business of the world.

Tennis star Jimmy Connors remarked, "In the past I found it hard to play well when my outside life wasn't going well, but now I have separated the two. I play tennis, and I have my family. I don't let either interfere with the other."

(In an entry that follows, "Mental Preparation," we will discuss this further.)

Concentration becomes a little more complex when the student or executive enters the classroom or conference room. Others in the room may be either critical or contentious. At the site of competition the weekend athlete must contend with opponents and perhaps spectators who may be distracting. This can be avoided if you have considered the kind of game (or questions) that your opponent will field. This you do in developing your strategy (see "Game Plan").

During the game you also have to cope with distractions that come at you without warning and usually without a label marked "Distraction." The most common distractions include:

—A wrinkle in your sock
—A fantastic shot made by your opponent
—The beginning of a blister
—The loss of a crucial point
—Concern about your conditioning
—The game lasting longer than you anticipated
—Missing a meeting or dinner
—Tiring out faster than your opponent
—The clock running fast

The above and several hundred other possible distractions may lead to a breakdown of concentration and loss of performance and game.

The fact is indisputable. No one can think of two things at the same time, and it may be another million years before the human brain has evolved to that level of function. In the meantime, accept the notice that there is no substitute for concentration.

The following suggestions should help:

1. Plan your strategy before the game. Make any changes during time-outs or when retrieving a ball. Once action begins, think only of the play.

2. If you are having equipment or clothing problems, call time and fix it.

3. If you are getting a blister, stop and tape it.

4. Agree with your opponent on a time to end the game, and when the time arrives, stop playing.

5. Keep your eye on the ball. If your eye begins to wander, try to tell which way the ball is spinning or look for the trademark. The rule applies no matter how tough your opponent.

Connors talking about John McEnroe noted, "He's a great server, even his second serve is tough, but I've learned to watch the ball closely."

6. Don't let a crucial point distract you.

Connors again: "Big points? They're all the same to me. I try not to panic at any time, no matter what the score. I stay calm at all times regardless of where I stand."

7. Maintain your condition so that fatigue won't be a problem.

8. Instantly block out any distraction that occurs on the side-lines or in the game. Pirate John Milner, after surviving a knock-down pitch to hit a grand-slam home run on the next pitch, said, "I've had closer calls than that. It didn't break my concentration."

9. Go into the game to win. Strive to win. If you are up against a better player, strive to be a tough competitor. All this is good for arousal and the maintaining of concentration.

10. Remember the words of Phil Mahre, world-class slalom skier, "You can't let up for a tenth of a second."

Confidence During the 1979 baseball season Pirate pitcher John Candelaria said, "They [the Orioles] could beat us the next twenty games in a row, and they're still not a better team than we are."

Although the World Series proved Candelaria's confidence to be well founded, his statement appears to be brash, typical of some athletes, but not really definitive. Athletic confidence puzzles a lot of people, especially those weekenders who are newcomers to competition.

Americans prefer the confidence of the "quiet man," the strong, silent demeanor of the John Waynes and Robert Redfords. There is nothing more impressive than a person who has earned confidence and nothing more degrading than empty confidence. We respect the quiet confidence of the person who has done his homework. We want to cry for the one who believes that an air of confidence can make up for laziness and incompetence.

In day-to-day living, confidence is our security blanket. We depend on it for peace of mind. Dentists, physicians, mechanics, and our families earn our trust through their competency. Furthermore, we expect to find confidence in others, even demand it. Would you board a 747 if the pilot doubted his ability to make a safe landing?

For ourselves, we prefer tasks that we are confident we can handle, not because we are afraid that we will fail but because we value our integrity, which in turn demands that we be responsible for our actions. We cannot accept responsibility confidently when we are uncertain of our capacity for a job.

An engineer would never think of presenting a design to the boss if there were a 50–50 chance that the engine would blow up.

A hostess would never prepare a special dish for guests if she were only half sure the recipe was dependable.

Then how can athletic opponents be so positive, so cocksure, when only one of the two can win the game?

This question confounds the nonathlete, but the explanation is simple. The true competitor, a Roger Bannister, for example, seeks out a challenge or is routinely confronted by challenge, as in the case of the scheduled athlete who goes from game to game until the season is completed. In facing up to a challenge, you are explicitly accepting the possibility of failure. This is the challenge to the human spirit that Bannister recognized, which in turn sharpens the senses to the level of exhilaration. No one has defined athletic confidence better than basketball player Willis Reed: "You always know you can lose, but you always think you're going to win."

For the weekend athlete, confidence must be rooted in proper conditioning and the practice of skills. Real confidence will not desert you if you get a bad break during a game, and it does not depend on winning.

Confidence may relate to the level of competition. When your opponent is clearly a superior player, set realistic goals. Decide before the game the number of points that you may reasonably expect to score. Sometimes you may win the game. That happens when the better player is overconfident.

Overconfidence frequently results in the player's not being aroused, not being mentally prepared, not arriving with a game plan or not concentrating.

Real confidence is always based on the reality of competition. Only a great athlete can say confidently, "You always know you can lose, but you always think you're going to win."

Daughters   Overcome psychosocial bias. Play ball with daughters. Penn State psychologist Dr. Dorothy Harris asserts, "Whatever it is that works for little boys also works for little girls." Treat daughters as you would sons. Make them compete. Make them chase balls, work hard, and stay in condition. They'll love you for it. Maybe.

Discipline   Bobby Knight, Indiana University's basketball coach, said, "My eight years at West Point allowed me not only an appreciation of discipline but also to find a way discipline could be applied to basketball and to the players I would coach. . . . I felt that West Point had prepared me for whatever I might encounter elsewhere. The atmosphere at the Academy and the people I met while coaching there gave me a background that I could not have obtained anywhere else."

Evaluation   Ernest Vandeweghe, M.D., former basketball star and father of Keke, "I have played a great deal in my career and never found losing better than winning."

Excellence, Striving For   Weekenders often have the wrong slant on excellence because many of us have had bad experiences with our parents and coaches during our childhood. As youngsters we are actually discouraged from sports competition by adults who demand that we reach for an unrealistic level of performance when in fact few of us can ever expect to hit a ball like Jack Nicklaus or John McEnroe.

In our opinion, excellence is making the best of your athletic talent and enjoying it. For the weekend athlete, no matter what your performance, you can find a game with someone at your level of play, and you both will enjoy the competition.

Follow the guidelines in this book for reaching your own level of excellence. Expect your children to strive for excellence, to do their best, but don't turn them off from sport by demanding that they play like champions.

Failure   John Neff, former high school coach at New Lexington, Ohio, and football mentor to James L. Anderson, quarterback, put failure and success in perspective when he said, "Success is not final, just as failure is not fatal."

Over the past twenty years a number of psychologists have warned us that failure is debilitating, especially for children. They forget that failure is a learning experience, that no one is successful all the time.

At West Point, and other colleges that have high admission standards, we see bright high school students who are almost always crushed when they arrive. They are no longer the only high achiever, number one in their class. Those who survive, who come back strong and confident, are usually the youngsters who have had athletic experience. They have learned that in life you win some and lose some. They have learned to use that failure to remind them to make a greater effort the next time. They have learned that life is worth living when you try your best.

Adults who are learning sports for the first time must grasp the win-lose psychology of sports. They must also come to appreciate the valuable experience that sports participation offers their children (see "Losers and Winners").

Fair Play   At the 1964 Winter Olympics, Eugenio Monti sacrificed international acclaim to the principle of fair play. In the two-man bobsled trials the Italian champion moved his team into first place. Only the sled piloted by Tony Nashathe, the English champion, had a chance of beating him. Word came to Monti at the base of the run that the Englishman would have to default because of a defective part in his sled. Monti detached the part from his sled and sent it up to Nashathe, who then beat Monti's time and won the Olympic gold medal.

Some praised Monti. Some found his act incomprehensible. Others said that Monti had made a grand gesture that backfired. A few thought that he should have his head examined. An American youngster out of the Midwest would have said that Monti was the kind of person who liked to win fair and square. Most children would understand Monti. Children play fairly without the help of umpires and referees.

Eugenio Monti received the first trophy awarded by the International Pierre de Coubertin Fair Play Trophy Committee. With the help of the committee's charter we would like to define fair play in a world where there appears to be some confusion about its meaning.

Fair play implies the sincere desire to base a win solely on performance. It refutes the principle of victory at any price and requires the strict observance of both the written and unwritten rules of sports.

The unwritten rules demand something more than being a good sport. Fair play is an exacting moral standard which advocates that to win by cheating or because of an umpire error or by an unfair stroke of fate is not really to win. Fair play involves accepting the risk that a fair play decision may affect the outcome of competition.

A weekender's attitude toward fair play may be somewhat compromised by the cynicism that surrounds scheduled athletics today. The excesses that we see give sports a bad name. However, we should remember that despite occasional reports of cheating and the arguments with umpires, athletes judge each other on ability. For the weekend athlete, fair play should be even more important because we play for the pure joy of the game. Therefore, choose your partners and opponents with care.

When you play against someone who takes advantage of line calls and does cute things to annoy you, your concentration falters, and zest is replaced by anger. If you continue to be scrupulously honest against such an opponent, he may be unnerved, but he's more likely to think that you're a damned fool. And you are if you continue to play with him.

Fatigue   Vince Lombardi: "Fatigue makes cowards of us all."

The Lombardi quote is fascinating. No one knew that he could sound like Shakespeare, and only his close friends appreciated his perceptions. Although he is remembered as a great strategist, a great teacher, and a great motivator, he also understood that confidence on the playing field was not solely dependent on desire but that the inner spirit itself depends on the absence of fatigue and the presence of vigor.

Most of us can put aside the tough decisions at the end of the day. We accept our fatigue and pick up our work in the morning. When we don't have the benefit of time and rest, the outcome is doubtful. An extreme example was observed during the Korean War, when poorly conditioned soldiers had to keep moving to avoid being captured or killed. Although their lives were on the line, many soldiers gave up because of fatigue. If a person can give up in a life-or-death situation, it can happen in a game and affect the outcome.

As fatigue begins to take over during competition, we worry about it, wonder if our opponent is also getting tired. We lose our concentration and begin to modify our game plan. We worry about missing the tough shots. We lose our psychological edge because we have lost our physiological edge.

Successful people know the importance of being awake on the job, but they don't always understand that it is also important for the weekend competitor. The conditioning program in this book is designed to develop your stamina and muscular endurance—and it will serve you at work and at play.

Frustration   A 5-year-old told his parents, "I threw away my bat because it didn't hit the ball."

Every athlete knows frustration. Reggie goes into a batting slump. Martina can't punch the corner. They score A plus in technique, ability, health, and motivation, but everything goes wrong. There is no accounting for their frustration. Weekend athletes also suffer frustration. We get out on the courts or the golf course, and we can't do what we are capable of doing. Like the 5-year-old, we want to throw away our racquets and clubs.

During competition, frustration leads to a loss of concentration, which in turn leads to more frustration, to anger, then apathy, and perhaps even aggression toward an opponent. Tennis player Ilie

Nastase reached that stage, and some weekend athletes get there. It's a bad scene.

When nothing works for you in competition, when you know that you are frustrated, accept it. That is a positive step. Work on your concentration. Change your strategy, and perhaps that will force your opponent to change his. If nothing works, remind yourself that no one plays at his peak all the time. Hold onto your confidence. Remember that tomorrow is another day.

When Tom Seaver pulled out of one of the worst slumps in his career, he said, "You can't escape slumps, but I never doubted myself."

A teammate, catcher Don Werner, observed, "The key was he never gave in."

Game Plan   Dominate is not a chauvinistic word in sports. Dominate means controlling the play, and that's why coaches put so much importance on a game plan. At the college and professional level, game planning is a complicated job that requires a host of people and things ranging from scouts to a late-generation computer. For the weekend athlete, however, it need be neither complicated nor time-consuming.

If you have only a few minutes, perhaps while you are walking from the dressing room to the court, you can develop a game plan, and it will give you a competitive edge. We'll use tennis as an example, although similar analysis and planning may be applied to any other sport.

If you've played your opponent or watched your opponent play, you're in luck. Begin by analyzing her or his weak and strong points—i.e., in poor condition, weak backhand, never comes to the net, seldom hits down the line, but very quick, strong serve, good forehand, almost always hits cross court.

Next, analyze your own play. Determine how to use your strong points and take advantage of your opponent's weaknesses. Perhaps you may decide to concentrate on your return of serve to be sure that you keep the ball in play. You will want to rely on a mix of short shots to draw your opponent to the net so that you can lob to the back of the court and thus force your opponent to run. You'll try to play to the backhand as much as possible. When you come to the net, you'll be prepared for a cross-court return.

During the warm-up, practice some of the shots that are involved in your game plan so that you will feel comfortable with your strategy when the game begins. Try to start strong to get an early advantage. Your opponent may panic.

If you don't know your opponent's game, go with your strong points at the start. If it goes well, continue with the plan until your opponent finds a way to counter. Then take a time-out, or during a changeover decide on a new strategy.

Game plans are not infallible. If you listen to big-time coaches after a loss, they usually explain that the opposition forced them to abandon their game plan. Perhaps they didn't have a good alternate plan. Perhaps they would have been outplayed under any circumstances. Still, when opponents are evenly matched, a game plan is almost always the key to victory.

Caution: Decide on your game plan before you get to the court, before the warm-up. Furthermore, never think about adjusting your strategy while the ball is in play. Don't try to analyze why you blew the last point or how you will play the next point even though it may be critical. Learn the discipline of concentrating only on the ball.

Hunger   See "Arousal."

John Wayne   Advising Kirk Douglas: "Guys like us gotta play strong parts." See "True Grit."

Joy   Pete Rose: "I have so much fun playing baseball. That's why I play the way I do."

La Gioconda Smile   A facial expression developed by Mona Lisa during overtime when she didn't want her opponent to discover that she was exhausted.

Losing and Losers   Ohio State's Woody Hayes once said, "You show me a good loser, and I'll show you a loser."

Very strong. Very macho. But the acceptability of the statement depends on the interpretation. For starters, it is very important to understand that losing does not have to make you a loser. In sports competition, no more than 50 percent of the participants can win. If professionals do that well, they will have their contracts renewed and perhaps even earn bonuses.

Normally sports experts use the 50 percent level as a sign of a successful season. In the National Basketball Association, a team with a 50 percent won-lost record will make the play-offs. In the National Hockey League, because of the prevalence of tie scores, less than 50 percent of the teams will win more than they lose. In major competition in golf, tennis, skiing, and ice skating, only one wins, but the others still rank among the world's greatest athletes. Certainly, you would think twice before calling any of them losers.

We are suggesting that you put losing in the proper context. Still, we should never shrug off losing. The disappointment should be a catalyst. Every loss should make you resolve to improve your conditioning and skill.

Perhaps Red Blaik said it better than Woody Hayes: "There is a big difference between a good sport and a good loser."

Luck   If you begin to play beyond your ability, enjoy it. Grin at your opponent, and tell him, "I'd rather be lucky than good." He may be superstitious and believe you.

Mental Preparation/Putting on Your Game Face   No matter how great their physical condition, scheduled athletes know that you must be mentally up to win a game. The pro, world-class, and college athletes have coaches and trainers working on their mental edge. Weekend athletes must do it on their own. Scheduled athletes may have days, weeks, or even months to get primed. The weekend athlete must do it in minutes.

The weekender should be able to spare at least twenty minutes in mental preparation. This may be the time that you spend in transportation and in changing clothes for the game. The secret is to stop thinking about work and problems the moment that you leave your home or office. That's when you begin putting on your game face. But you must be alone.

If a colleague, friend, or spouse decides to walk or ride you to the club to keep you company, to discuss business or a domestic matter, you will subsequently find it difficult to concentrate during the game. Of course, the same problem exists if you are alone and think about your next business appointment, the work on your desk, or the chores that are waiting for you at home.

In addition to preparing a game plan during this period, you must find a way to get pumped up to your best level of performance. You may have to experiment with different ways of going about this. It may be remembering the last time that you lost to your opponent and then resolving not to let it happen again. Or it may be placing a friendly bet with your opponent or merely recalling how good it feels when you play your very best. One weekender told us that he occasionally promises himself a new T-shirt if he wins. But keep at it until you develop those butterflies (see "Arousal").

Never think of anything else but the game if you want to win. That's the simplicity of mental preparation.

Mixed Doubles Women should never play with male chauvinists. However, it's okay if male chauvinists play with female chauvinists. They deserve each other.

Opponents Given the opportunity, weekend athletes should choose opponents according to their level of play.

The most competitive level is normally between evenly matched opponents. However, losing to someone who is your equal may be the most difficult to accept, although it shouldn't be. Theoretically you should win about 50 percent of the time.

When we play someone who is clearly our superior—and many of us enjoy doing that occasionally—we play harder, play better to keep up our end, and may also learn something. Still, there's a pitfall to be avoided. When we lose to a better player, we can tell ourselves and others that we could not expect to win. The player who chooses a superior player as an opponent most of the time should consider his motives. He may be afraid to win and so assures a loss. This kind of player does not want the responsibility of being a winner.

Competing with an inferior has specific problems. If you play your best, you know that you will win; if you take it easy, you may lose your concentration and then hand your opponent the classic underdog advantage. This may be a trying situation.

We talked to a West Point wife who complained that her husband let her win points. Her husband, a former varsity tennis player and a tough competitor, didn't know what to do. He couldn't refuse to play with her and hurt her feelings. On the other hand, if he played tough, she seldom scored and wound up frustrated.

For a time he tried giving her a handicap, although he didn't like the idea because he believes that the handicapped competitor begins a game with a negative attitude. He gave her first a 30-love handicap and then 40-love. However, she was gutsy and objected. So they had arrived at an impasse.

There's no moral to the story, but it makes a point. If competition is going to be mentally satisfying, opponents must be fairly matched, not selected on the basis of love or affection.

Over 30   Tennis star Billie Jean King: "People think when you reach 30 that you're through. Well, I'll tell you something. I'm going to be moving a whole lot faster when I'm 65 than people who are 30 who think that way."

Paying the Price   After logging his three thousandth base hit, Boston's Carl Yastrzemski said, "I haven't had the greatest ability in the world. I'm not a big strong guy. I've made nine million changes, nine million adjustments. I've worked hard during the wintertime. I've paid the price."

At West Point we always remember Col. Earl "Red" Blaik, the Academy's most successful football coach (1941 to 1958). During this period Blaik won three national championships with three undefeated seasons; his players won seven Lambert trophies, and thirty-six were elected to the all-American first team. However, the heritage that Red Blaik left us was the maxim he coined: "You have to pay the price." He told us that a winner must work hard, practice arduously, and maintain self-discipline. We apply this to academics, sports, and military education.

Doc Counsilman, who has twice coached the U.S. Men's Olympic swimming team, including the 1972 team that starred Mark Spitz, puts paying the price another way with his "Hurt, Pain, Agony Theory." Counsilman believes that the difference between the normally talented and the world-class athlete is a matter of accepting escalating degrees of pain:

Normally talented athletes will practice until they are fatigued and their muscles begin to *hurt*; at that point they feel that they must stop, and they do.

World-class athletes drive themselves beyond the *hurt* threshold and continue to work until the body is in real *pain* and then stop.

World-class champions pass through the hurt and pain threshold until their bodies are in *agony*. They accept the *agony*, drive longer and harder through the *agony* until they win.

Olympic swimmer Brian Job observes, "There's always a fear. You know you're not going to die, but you know if you swim a fast time, it will hurt so much, and you're afraid of that."

Steven Prefontaine, an American premier distance runner, said, "A lot of people run a race to see who is the fastest. I run to see who has the most guts, who can punish himself into an exhausting pace, and then at the end who can punish himself even more. Pain tolerance is a prerequisite for championship performance."

We honor world champions for their skills and superb conditioning, but we should also honor the price that they are willing to pay. By contrast, the weekender's cost is very small—perhaps thirty minutes of mild conditioning a day. Still, the weekender should be conscientious and disciplined, and accept the stress principle in order to improve performance. And paying the price applies equally to women weekenders.

Dr. Joanna Davenport, professor and director of women's athletics at Auburn University, a visiting professor at West Point and a tough competitor on the courts, says, "Women respect the principle of paying the price in most areas of their lives. A mother doesn't give up on a child who makes an error. She doesn't give up on any moral principle that is worth fighting for. It's a way of life that is not only human but wholesome. But paying the price also means that if you lose the first set, you must be tough and come back."

And paying the price applies equally to any age-group. It is never too late to shape up, as Doc Counsilman proved before his 1979 swim across the English Channel at age 58. However, Doc

Counsilman takes a modest view of his feat and places it in the lowest threshold of pain.

He says, "It only hurt once—from the beginning to the end."

Peak Performance Peak performance is as much mental as physical, so uniquely sensational that it has the impact of a phenomenon. It is so exhilarating that weekenders talk about peak performance in wondering tones. The experience is known to professional, amateur, and weekend athletes, both youngsters and adults.

The body is exceptional during a peak performance. Concentration is nearly 100 percent, so nearly perfect that the ball appears to be standing still and as big as a full moon when you meet it. Coordination and timing are perfect, and you win with a kind of ease that is almost euphoric.

You can't predict when or how frequently you will experience this wonderful unity of body and mind, but there are several factors that must be present. You must be physically and mentally prepared. And you must be playing against a tough competitor who pumps you up. You will easily beat your opponent, but he or she will understand what's happened because peak performance is solely the experience of the tough competitor.

Playing Not To Lose In tennis, it is called becoming tentative; in other sports, losing momentum. We go up against a superior player expecting to lose. Instead of playing to win, we play not to lose. Or we fall behind in evenly matched competition, become defensive, and play not to lose. It is a very common syndrome, and a bad one. The psychology is all wrong.

Mike Krzynzewski, West Point basketball coach, once said, "We want our kids to play to their potential, to feel good about themselves. Of course, we want to win all our games, but what we really want to know is that every time we walk off the court, we can look at each other and say, 'Hey, we played our butts off out there.' If we lose to a team that's superior, well, they have to beat us. We don't want to beat ourselves."

If you play not to lose, you beat yourself (see "Arousal" and "Confidence").

Psyching Gamesmanship known as psyching is stupid and sick. Psyching out someone means disturbing an opponent emotionally and is often practiced by those who appear to be emotionally disturbed. Psych artists usually psych themselves out or psych up their opponents with their crass attempts.

Quality Fred M. Hechinger, education specialist and member of *The New York Times* editorial board: "Excellence and competition are no longer the dirty words they came to be in the 1960's."

Remembrance In the 1978 World Series, the late Thurman Munson played with a separated shoulder, his throwing arm grinding and groaning, but he threw out the Dodgers' best basestealers. He was able to do this, he later explained, "because I wanted to do it." Munson was always a tough competitor. He once said, "I could never approach a baseball game or a business deal with less than 100 percent effort."

Risk Taking The question of when to go after a low percentage shot often makes the difference between winning and losing. The risk entails taking a calculated gamble at the key point in a match rather than waiting for your opponent to hit a winner or make a mistake.

Risk taking should not be suicidal. That is, you should risk only a strategy that you have practiced, that you have a chance of pulling off. You should consider taking a risk under certain circumstances:

> —When you are playing a superior opponent and the game is up for grabs.
> —If you can win with the risk but not jeopardize your chances if the risk fails.
> —If your game plan is working and you want to put additional pressure on your opponent.
> —If your game plan is working and you want to demonstrate your ability to maintain confidence.

Of course, the calculated risk should be used sparingly and never be considered part of the whole strategy in your game plan.

Furthermore, you should begin to get some familiarity with risk-taking strategy. Give it some practice when playing an inferior opponent and you are safely ahead.

Sleep	A good night of it is helpful in maintaining concentration.

Sportsmanship	Leo Durocher: "Nice guys finish last."
Fair play and sportsmanship are not synonymous. An act of fair play means assigning a point to your opponent that may affect the outcome of a game. Sportsmanship is concerned with etiquette, concern for your opponent's well-being, dignity in defeat, and grace in victory. Being a nice guy is an important factor in the enjoyment of competition. Being a nice guy is altogether compatible with being a tough competitor. Durocher is wrong.

Teamwork	Team games are valuable during a youngster's formative years. The child develops leadership but also learns to work for a common goal and sacrifice individual glory for the good of the group. These are the same qualities that an adult should look for in choosing a tennis partner or picking up a soccer team.

Tenacity	Ara Parseghian, former head coach at Notre Dame "We always outmanned West Point, but I always admired their fitness and tenacity."

True Grit	Martina Navratilova, remembering the years before she became a world tennis champion, recalled: "Everybody said I was crazy. I was losing, losing, losing, but still I was attacking."

Winning	You cannot become a winner unless you compete.

Winning Words	"O the glory of the winning . . ."—George Meredith.
Cicero relates that Diagoras, who won a prize at Olympia and then witnessed two sons' being crowned on the same day, was honored by a speech that began: "Die, Diagoras, for thou has nothing short of divinity to desire."
The New York Times relates that Steeler Coach Chuck Noll,

after witnessing his team winning the Super Bowl for the third time, told the Steelers, "You haven't yet reached your peak."

And what goes on in the mind of the victor?

When reporters asked a Sherpa mountain climber what he was thinking of when he reached the peak of Mount Everest, he replied, "How to get down."

Index